CONTENTS

Stronger Together

How We're Living While Fighting

LINDA & ANNE NOLAN

with Sarah Robertson

EBURY
PRESS

1 3 5 7 9 10 8 6 4 2

Ebury Press, an imprint of Ebury Publishing
20 Vauxhall Bridge Road
London SW1V 2SA

Ebury Press is part of the Penguin Random House group of companies
whose addresses can be found at global.penguinrandomhouse.com

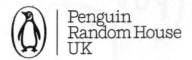

This book is a work of non-fiction based on the life, experiences
and recollections of the author. In some cases, names of people,
places, dates, sequences and the detail of events have been
changed to protect the privacy of others.

First published by Ebury Press in 2021
This paperback edition is published in 2022

www.penguin.co.uk

A CIP catalogue record for this book is available from the British Library

ISBN 9781529109597

Printed and bound in Great Britain by Clays Ltd, Elcograf S.p.A.

The authorised representative in the EEA is Penguin Random House Ireland,
Morrison Chambers, 32 Nassau Street, Dublin D02 YH68

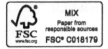

Penguin Random House is committed to a
sustainable future for our business, our readers
and our planet. This book is made from Forest
Stewardship Council® certified paper.

PROLOGUE

PROLOGUE

FEBRUARY 2020

There's a scene in the film *Titanic* where the character of older Rose, played by the late Gloria Stuart, describes how the ill-fated vessel was named by some the 'Ship of Dreams'.

We could relate to that feeling of pure joy and excitement when we boarded the MSC *Grandiosa* on 28 February of last year, to embark on our own dream adventure sailing on the high seas.

For the first time in our adult lives, we four sisters had found ourselves single; so when a TV company asked us to come on board one of the biggest cruise ships in the world and sing again for a new eight-part reality show called *The Nolans Go Cruising* on digital channel Quest Red, well, we couldn't say no to our own TV show together.

Joined by Coleen, 55, and Maureen, 66, we were queens of the world as we floated around the Mediterranean on a luxurious liner, feeling like royalty and living the high life with not a care or worry beyond planning our holiday outfits and preparing for a performance of our biggest hit, 'I'm In The Mood For Dancing', in front of our fellow passengers on the final night of the trip.

From five-star-level wining and dining to visiting incredible European destinations, the entire experience was the holiday of a lifetime.

And as Nolan fans well know, us siblings have endured many public feuds over the years, so we can't blame them if they initially thought this wasn't going to be plain sailing, wondering – with four very different woman all bundled together in one place 24/7 for two weeks – how long it would take for them to hit the waves and be shipwrecked.

Even we had a teeny bit of concern that old wounds might be sliced back open, while Coleen, the youngest of us, publicly voiced her fears that there was a chance that after the show we could end up getting off the cruise ship and never speaking to each other again.

It's likely that Maureen, like ourselves, was also feeling slightly apprehensive; having worked in the public eye and dealt with the media for years, we know they love a row as it makes great telly.

But fortunately for our sibling relationship, the opposite happened. It was smooth sailing all the way and with no horrible stories or arguments on or off camera; we simply reconnected as a family, and it may sound a little corny or clichéd, but the love really did overflow during the holiday. We became the closest as sisters we had been since first breaking into the world of pop music as a band nearly 50 years ago.

But as we danced up a storm together night after night at the ship's disco while rejoicing in our good fortune, enjoying glasses of champagne while laughing and joking about little silly crushes on some of the handsome men we had seen on our travels, little did we know that we were about to be swept away by a storm of tsunami proportions that would test any family.

The first waves of the coronavirus pandemic were beginning to cause a ripple, but that was not the sinister disease that was to turn our worlds upside down, although it has brought its own kind of misery and suffering.

No, it was not Covid-19 creating havoc in our bodies, but another insidious disease running amok inside us both – cancer.

Cancer has blighted and haunted the Nolan family for more than 20 years, robbing us of our beloved sister Bernie at only 52.

So, when we found out it had come for both of us at the same time, we decided to team up and fight it all the way together as sisters, because we are stronger together.

This story is about how the unbreakable bond and strength of sisterly love and female friendship has helped us deal with the raw blows and curveballs life has thrown at both of us over the last two decades.

It's not a diary as such as we are rubbish at remembering dates! But each chapter explores our journey dealing cancer and the experiences we have shared along the way as sisters and a family, mixed with a dollop of good old Nolan humour and wisdom.

We also address universal issues relating to cancer, such as losing your hair, and how we managed to deal with the unpleasant side effects cancer treatment gives you.

5

You may have picked up this book having just been diagnosed with cancer yourself or know someone with it, or perhaps just want to read about two women who tell it like it is. And while this is not a self-help book and we are not offering any medical advice or claiming special knowledge, we hope you find it helpful and it brings you some comfort to know that, if you're facing adversity, you're not alone in your struggles.

All our love,

Anne and Linda X

CHAPTER 1

THE CALM BEFORE THE STORM

ANNE

At one stage it was touch and go whether we would make it on board the ship last February. Italy was one of the first European countries to be hit badly by the emerging Covid pandemic, and we were supposed to be boarding the *Grandiosa* in Genoa in northern Italy.

But an outbreak of coronavirus in the Italian city put paid to that plan and the programme's producers were forced to divert their schedule at the last minute.

It was an anxious wait to hear if our route could be changed with just hours to go, and after a tense few hours, we were given the all-clear to embark and set sail.

We would like to say that no one had any idea at that stage how serious things would get with the pandemic. When we were waiting to board the ship last year, the World Health Organization hadn't even referred to it as a pandemic. And in fact, they didn't declare it as one until 11 March, by which point our holiday was nearly over.

This sailing trip was the first time the four of us had properly been together 24/7 in about 20 years, and we all wanted it to go well for so many different reasons.

As sisters we wanted to help Linda find love because she had been through such a tough time having lost Brian, her husband, and then being told in 2017 that she had secondary cancer in her hip. But, if I'm being honest, I think all of us were a little nervous at first about what to expect being thrown in the deep end together for that length of time, because there is no proper escape when you are on board a ship, despite its mammoth size. It's not like one of you can say, right, I've had enough of you all, then get in the car and drive off to your own home!

Therefore, some of that trepidation before we went on the show was about having arguments.

We all have our own personalities – even the quiet ones like me have our moments – and all of us were thinking, Oh God, are we going to last these two weeks? And also – I cannot swim!

Before we went on the cruise, I think each of us individually thought, let's try to not let things get to each of us if they do; my thinking was that anything annoying will be about little things, rather than anything major. When I look back, I think that's what we all did.

I thought, if somebody is getting on my nerves or they say something that I'm not happy with, then I'm going to let it go over my head and not allow it to get to me.

However, any silly fears we may have harboured soon dissipated and it was just wonderful that nothing like that happened. It was so carefree and happy that we were all getting on so well.

It was a carefree, fantastic, and happy time, which I think came across in the programme on TV, about which we had so much good feedback.

If I were asked to describe the overriding emotion I felt on the holiday, it would be one of joy. The atmosphere was warm and inviting, and we all felt uplifted in each other's company.

We drank together, ate out as a family together, we worked together, rehearsed for the grand finale reunion show, and visited the most amazing, beautiful cities and towns, meeting some incredible people, all side by side – I never wanted the holiday to end.

The ship was beautiful, and it was five-star treatment and luxury all the way.

We all had our own cabins equipped with bathrooms and balconies you could sit out on and watch the waves as you crossed the water. It was fabulous.

When asked whether being filmed prevented us from enjoying our experience on board, the answer is no.

The television crew were simply amazing. I forgot we were being filmed, that's how discreet they were.

I think it's also why the series came across so naturally, because we forgot we were being filmed and nothing was rehearsed.

The crew was very relaxed and simply suggested ideas for what they would like us to do, or where they wanted us to go, and the rest was just us four being ourselves.

Also, it didn't feel like we were being set up when we were being filmed for the show, unlike some reality shows where they seem to place the participants in scenes where they will squabble and fall out. There was nothing like that with us and the producers told us, 'If you say something and then you change your mind, because you didn't like the way it came out, then absolutely say.'

Hearing that, we felt protected, and we talked about what we wanted. There was no rehearsing of lines or saying, let's try this and let's do that.

We were unaware they were filming us.

And only once or twice did they ask us to walk our steps again because of lighting issues.

We just went ahead and were ourselves, warts, and all. When I watched it back last summer, I was so pleased with it because of how natural it was.

During the trip we did a lot of reminiscing about things that had happened, stuff that was bad, and other things that were now good in our lives.

I think the bond I now have with my sisters – with all my sisters – is unbreakable.

It was nearly broken years ago in the fallout over a past reunion tour, after which we didn't speak for three years.

But now there is absolutely nothing that would make me do something that might estrange me from my sisters again. We've never fallen out since and visiting all these countries and places together was a lesson in how we are so much happier and better when we are together. I would never let anything break us apart again ever.

The holiday was also a great time for me to connect with Linda. She had already been through a storm at the time of us going away together.

She had been diagnosed three years earlier with secondary cancer in her hip, was suffering with arthritis, lymphoedema in her arm and has also battled depression following the loss of her beloved husband Brian.

Yet, she's always smiling and doing her best to cheer others up. We wanted to do something nice for her, and there was a glorious afternoon we spent together thanks to Coleen, who had booked Linda and me into the spa to have some pampering massages.

Skin glowing and feeling blissed out, we wandered up to the top deck afterwards in our white robes to continue our happy vibe lying on the sun loungers, sipping a cocktail each and relaxing.

We started talking about our original cancer battles and how fortunate we felt to have come through them. I had been given the all-clear from breast cancer in 2005 and Linda had been free of breast cancer for nearly a decade, and, while she had been dealing with the secondary cancer in her hip for a few years, it seemed to be under control.

During our catch-up Linda opened up to me quite deeply about her body issues with the lymphoedema in her arm and the scars and how they have affected her confidence.

I have thankfully never really suffered from that issue. I mean, when I was young I thought I had big ears and bony knees, which I did and which I still do, but as I got older, I thought, oh God, you know, if somebody is going to have a go at me because

I've got big ears and bony knees, well, they've got more problems than I have. And I just got to that stage where I thought, I do not care. If I'm fine with it, and other people are not, well, that's their problem, not mine. I told Linda this, and she said, I know, Anne, but it does still worry me.

Because Linda has such a friendly personality and disposition – she is what you would call an extrovert – I didn't realise the extent to which it had been affecting her. For example, she would not get undressed or go in the swimming pool in front of strangers. And while she was carrying on and happy in the present time, she still had body issues, which were giving her angst.

We went back to our cabins to get ready for cocktails and dinner, and I reflected on how much I'd enjoyed that lovely afternoon with my sister putting the world to rights and being close to her.

Looking back on that day now, it was the calm before the storm – the real story building up was back on dry land. At the start of our trip I was pottering around in my cabin and flipped the news on the TV, where it flashed up there had been 12 Covid cases in Britain. Maureen mentioned it when we met up but at that point, while I thought 12 cases certainly was not something to be taken lightly, it also was not enough to stop me in my tracks, and I went about my day, not giving it that much thought.

But as we touched down in various places in Italy and Spain along the route we were taking we saw more and more people wearing masks or plastic visors and we thought, dear God, that's ridiculous, aren't they going over the top, because we were in this lovely bubble from sailing around on a cruise liner, and had no idea how bad it was getting.

To be fair we did always stay cautious and safe by religiously washing our hands and spritzing them with sanitiser.

Then, by the end of the cruise, the news reports on TV were saying the case number in the UK had shot up to 50, and we started to feel real concern about what was happening at home.

The ship's staff were fantastic and stayed on high alert, making sure passengers were sanitising hands, and we would have our temperatures checked when coming in and off the liner for our excursions, so we never felt in danger on our journey.

As the holiday drew to a close, we each started asking aloud what would happen when we arrived home?

Here we were, all together again, and none of us liked the idea of suddenly being separated and having to isolate for two weeks having been on this fantastic cruise.

As we had effectively been in a bubble together, Maureen suggested she and I stayed together at hers and then Linda would isolate in her own house and just come over to us at night for dinner because we had been together anyway. Coleen had gone home to Cheshire where she was isolating with her family.

Having gone out so much on holiday, we were suddenly no longer able to go out, and instead the kids and grandkids would be coming around to chat outside the window, passing signs and waving.

The isolation period at the very beginning was not all that bad. I may be the only one to think this, but I thought it quite nice because it was a novelty.

When the two weeks of isolation were up, I came home to my house, unaware my world and my family's was about to be turned upside down ...

LINDA

On the cruise ship life was carefree and glorious. We were thrilled to have been asked to do the show, but in the back of all our minds was the question: will it work – will we get on spending that much time together? But honestly, I could not have had a better time. I laughed so much, and we would end up every night in the *Grandiosa*'s Skyline Bar where the girls would have a cup of tea, but I, being a gin girl, would get stuck into the cocktail menu. I mean you can't go on holiday and not enjoy the all-inclusive bar!

Can you believe in my 60-something years, I had never had a full body massage before, so baby sister Coleen kindly decided to rectify this travesty and arranged a lovely surprise spa day for just me and Anne.

I feel a little bad thinking back to that morning because when Coleen said she and Maureen were going ashore in Italy to visit the town of Civitavecchia, outside of Rome, I got a bit fed up that Anne and I had been excluded and texted her, saying, why can't we go, too?

And she had to explain that it was because she had booked these massages as a surprise for Anne and me.

We both loved having those massages – oh they were lovely – and I can't believe I have missed out on having them all these years.

They put us in the same room – separate beds, of course! – and these two lovely masseuses from Thailand got to work, kneading out all our knots and muscle tension as we lay side by side.

The girls must have had magic fingers because it seemed like they had ironed out all my stresses and worries from my body and I just floated off the bed. I felt as light as a feather.

Wearing our robes and our skin covered in all these delicious-smelling oils and lotions, Anne suggested we go upstairs and get some fresh air and watch the sunset before meeting the rest of the gang for dinner.

We wandered together up to the top deck and on seeing the view, said to each other, 'is this not fabulous?'

I turned to Anne and said, 'Who'd have thought when I had my cancer that we would ever be able to do this kind of thing?', and Anne nodded in agreement, replying: 'Same here. Back then I thought, am I ever going to see my kids grow up?'

It was a very romantic view looking out to sea. So did Anne and I decide to re-enact Kate Winslet and Leo DiCaprio's famous scene in the movie, *Titanic*, where she goes, 'I'm flying, Jack!'?

Did we heck! No chance of that happening when we have a combined age of 131 – I mean, the *Titanic* hadn't even been built that long ago.

Instead, I decided to celebrate us being alive and winning against cancer in a much more delightful way, which was with a delicious sparkling glass of ice-cold champagne.

Who needs Leo anyway when you have a glass of bubbles and your big sister by your side?

Sitting down together, we talked about how well the holiday had gone and how we felt closer to each other. Anne is nine years older than me – a gap that felt bigger when we were growing up. When I was 11, she was 20, which is massive, and it does make a difference, but being on holiday brought us closer together, and by doing the stuff we did like having our massages and pampering days.

We laughed and spoke about our illnesses and I told her how my scars and body image was a big thing for me and that's why I actually had never had a full body massage before because I was self-conscious about my scars.

Talking about our lives together and having both been cancer survivors felt lovely and I loved getting closer to Anne.

'I remembered when I was told I had to have chemo, you were the first person I phoned because you had been there,' I told her.

I would ask her questions about the process and she would phone me up and give hints and tips such as if your taste buds go eat something very spicy or sweet.

It was all just friendly and loving, really. We spoke in depth about Bernie, and how Anne and I had both had breast cancer, but Bernie had lost her life to it. Without wanting to sound too cheesy – sorry in advance – do tell people you love them. Do not be frightened to let them know what they mean to you and make time to do the things you have been saying you are going to do.

How many times, if there is an old friend or relative, have you said, I must phone them because I haven't spoken to them in ages? Make the effort and do it, because one day it may be too late.

When we came off the ship and watched that episode back, Anne and I had just come out to the public about our cancer, so it was all over the news and in the papers, and a lot of people texted or tweeted after watching the show to say how bittersweet it was to watch us both feeling so good only for such tragedy to hit us again.

Our sister Denise also said afterwards, 'Oh, that was awful, seeing you both like that with what's happening now.'

It was definitely the most time we'd spent together since we were kids, because of our busy lives, our various tours, and Coleen doing her *Loose Women* show and TV work.

We filmed from seven in the morning until seven at night each day, and we had this group thing we always did at the end of each day. I called it a Cheers of the Day, where we would sit, with a cocktail sometimes, and toast our little family bubble.

It was lovely as were the pina coladas, which went down very well!

Also going down very well – or shall I say, what was very easy on the eye – were the gorgeous Italian men we kept meeting.

Everybody kept telling me before I set sail that I would be flirting with the captain; well, that never happened because, can you believe, we never met the bloody captain?

We were on an Italian ship with an Italian crew and we were meant to be having dinner with its captain when it stopped in Malta.

Sadly, due to some inclement weather in the Mediterranean, the captain had to reroute the whole ship so there was no time for dinner with the guests on that night.

But I did make up for it with some heavy-duty flirting with some of the other handsome men I met on our various excursions.

I flirted heavily with Salvatori, who was our tour guide during our time in Palermo.

He was a rather attractive 50-something bloke and very enjoyable to flirt with, but towards the end he mentioned to me his wife and children and I went, okay, byeee!

Men, eh? Still, Italian men flirt with their mothers, and it's always nice when anybody seems to pay you a little bit of attention.

The girls were laughing at me, saying those big saucer eyes of yours were staring up at him, Linda. I said, I am telling you now, he was flirting with me a little bit too. I found it hilarious.

The trouble is that in these situations you become 15 again – well, at least I did, because I could feel myself blushing furiously like I used to when I was a teenager, which was very embarrassing.

I admit I did give it some of the old Linda blue eyed flirty charm and batted my eyelashes at him – you never lose it!

When we arrived in Barcelona for Coleen's birthday on 12 March we were sitting down and one of the waiters came down and told me that Dimitri (one of the producers) wanted a word with me.

I was panicking that Salvatore might be upstairs. I told the girls, 'it won't be funny if he is actually up there', and turned into that awkward 15-year-old at the thought.

But I was not prepared for romance. I had no lipstick on, my face was tomato coloured from blushing, I was not wearing the right outfit I wanted to be seen in and generally just was not ready to go out on a date.

All this silly teenage crush nonsense was going around in my head and the girls pointed out I was physically shaking and sweating.

After all this, when I did pluck up the courage to go and meet Salvatori, he was nowhere to be seen. Dimitri had merely wanted me to go up and take part in a Zoom call with Coleen's son Shane Jr, unbeknownst to Coleen.

Why was I summoned to a call with Shane Jr? It happened that he was staying in another hotel in Barcelona, and was planning on surprising his mum for her birthday, and as my little treat to Coleen I had helped to arrange it.

More embarrassed that I raced upstairs thinking I was off to ride into the sunset with an Italian stallion, I realised how ridiculous I had been acting over the opposite sex and when I came back down, I told the others, 'I can't think of anything worse than dating. All this, what am I going to wear, where am I going to go … why do people put themselves through it?'

But the other people in the crew turned and declared online dating is brilliant because you spend time chatting online before going out for a drink and it cuts a lot of time wasting.

The girls put me on the dating app Tinder and everybody on the crew was going, Linda, Tinder is just for a quick shag, to which I was horrified.

Anne says she does not need male companions in the romantic sense in her life and sometimes I think I don't really need it either. Who can be bothered with somebody coming in and leaving a wet towel on the bed – not that I would sleep with him on the first date, of course – or making a mess in the house and putting things in the wrong place?

I've lived on my own for 13 years now, but I do think to be romanced and wined and dined would be lovely. That romantic flame in me is still glowing and has not gone out just yet. Maybe Anne and me should have a dating show; it would make great telly.

The highlight of the trip, though, was our relationships with each sister becoming rock solid. We spoke about it on the last night before we finished up the cruise. Still out at sea, we went to the bar to get some mocktails – we were going out to do something in the evening and had to stay alert – and reflected on our journey over the last 14 days.

I said to the other three that I felt the holiday really had worked and cemented our relationship to rock solid.

My life is much better with my sisters in it. We are a family and that's how it should be, and just sitting there together like we had been doing was the icing on the cake. The only thing that could have made it better was if our sister Denise, our two brothers – and Bernie, of course – could have been with us too.

The others agreed with me and we just spoke about what we learned about each other. I turned to Anne and said, 'I got closer to you. When I was ten you were twenty and going out with

Maureen and Denise, and I must have been this really annoying little sister.'

We hugged, and, in that moment, cancer was the furthest thing from my mind.

CHAPTER 2

THE
FIRST
TIME

LINDA

'I'm afraid it's cancer.'

There's news you want to receive in life, like you've won the lottery, Mrs Hudson, or you've got number one in the record charts, but sat in a hospital room being told you have cancer are not words you want to hear at any age, least of all when you are in the prime of your life, as I was the first time I got this thing.

People have asked me what goes through your mind when you get told that you have cancer. I tell them: dread. That is the only way to describe the feeling. Complete dread, followed by the unavoidable question: am I going to die?

That is why they put a Macmillan nurse in the room with you, I think. It's so they can do all the listening because your mind shuts down in shock, so when you go home and process it a little bit and regain your composure, you have somebody to call up and ask, er, what just happened in there? Along with all the other questions, like what do we do now, and when am I starting treatment?

I always say to people, if you are going to see your oncologist (that's a cancer specialist), just make sure you always have a note pad and a pen with you. And if you have got any questions that you want to ask, write them all down so you don't forget, and then write his or her answers down. Or bring a friend with you to do that for you or record it. The staff won't mind because, initially, it's so much information to take in.

The first time I was told I had cancer was back in 2006. To make sense of where I am now in my cancer story, I have to take you all back in time to the beginning. I was in Belfast playing the Wicked Queen in the panto, and I got the news of the results of my biopsy in between shows. Thinking back to that time brings up a whole array of emotions in me. I mean I'm scared of the dentist; Denise says to me, 'Every single thing you've been through in your life and you're still scared of the dentist.'

I got that feeling in my stomach – the butterflies of 'I don't want to go' and it was that kind of feeling all day on the Friday. I'd taken my stage make-up off before getting in the car with Brian because I couldn't have rocked up to the hospital looking like the Wicked Queen; otherwise they'd have put me in a different ward!

We drove to the hospital in silence. It was like the elephant in the room where up until that point, even though you both know the answer and are preparing yourself for the worst, there's a code of 'well, if we don't mention it then it won't happen', so we remained quiet.

We parked up and made our way to the ward where everything then speeded up. A nurse greeted us and led me to meet the doctor, who gently broke it to me that the biopsy showed it was breast cancer, which was stage three.

Certain words leapt out from the others as he continued explaining my diagnosis, such as chemotherapy, radiotherapy, and mastectomy. It felt surreal, and the closest thing I can liken it to was having some sort of out-of-body experience.

I think I must have zoned out because all that was going through my head as the doctor carried on talking was, this does not apply to me, this cannot be real, this is somebody else's news.

My insides were winded like I had been knocked hard sideways with a blunt instrument. I squeezed Brian's hand and looked across at him. He too looked like he had been hit by a stunning blow. Brian's face looked shocked as he absorbed what the doctor was telling both of us and he went completely white. His face looked so pale I thought he was going to faint and the nurse who was in the room obviously thought it too because she came over and gave him some water.

Trying to keep it together and remain calm, I told the consultant we would be flying back to England after the weekend.

Sadly, I can't recall this doctor's name, but he was very helpful and replied, 'Mrs Hudson, I will have all your notes ready for when you go back to your doctor, so you won't need another biopsy.'

When we finally stumbled out of that hospital room, Brian just turned to me and said, 'It's okay to cry now', and I just collapsed in his arms, sobbing, wondering what on earth I would do now.

On the way back to our digs in Belfast, I watched as people went about their everyday business. That was me just a few days earlier in my old pre-cancer life, I thought, when I was full of energy. I too was once that girl who was out shopping or working, travelling, not a care in the world, just busy making plans.

I think it was John Lennon who coined the adage, life is what happens to you while you're busy making other plans. Well, cancer was not on my list of things I needed to tick off that year or any year for that matter.

And then I thought of myself as being stupid because I had left my lump for so long.

You see, I knew I had a lump in my left breast, but instead of putting it to the top of my to-do list and calling up my GP to get it checked, I had left it for ages and ages and ages, a whole year to be exact.

When I was 20, I had a lump in the breast, which turned out to be a blocked milk duct.

At first I never told anybody about the new lump as I was busy working on the *Blood Brothers* tour and I just thought, ooh, bit of a lump there, but because I'd had a lump before, I never gave it any real thought.

Then, during the tour, we had a contract come up in Ireland for the panto over the winter season, which was great because it meant we had a steady income coming.

Brian had been undertaking treatment for skin cancer and I knew we needed this job. Eventually, though, the lump became too noticeable to ignore, and by the time I did go to the doctor in Belfast to have it sorted I was told the lump was 9cm by 5cm long. If you are not au fait with the sizes of breast lumps, in layman's terms it was massive.

The first thought that came into my head was: will I die? The other horrible thought going around my mind was: am I going to lose my hair? Terror set in as I thought of all the horror stories I had heard about chemotherapy.

I kept torturing myself, about how, if I had gone to the doctor straight away when I had first found it, things could be different.

I also had to break the terrible news to my family ...

My youngest sister Coleen was the one who I told first. Before I went to Belfast, I had told her about finding a lump and she had been nagging me daily, saying, 'Have you been to the doctor yet? If you do not see a doctor, then I am going to tell the others and they'll all be on the phone, saying have you been to the doctor?!'

Saying that I did have breast cancer out loud to Coleen made it all real and Brian came across and had to take the phone from me.

As I sat there crying, he spoke to Coleen, and she agreed she would tell the others about my cancer as it was becoming too much for me.

At this point, another thought was creeping into my head: what to do about work.

It may sound crazy that I was thinking about work at a shocking time like that, but, as they say in the entertainment business, the show must go on. There were three shows left to do in Belfast, and I was going back on that stage that evening, cancer, or no cancer.

Brian gently asked me, 'Lin, would you like me to phone them and tell them you can't come in?'

My look alone was enough to tell him that was a stupid idea.

But just in case he had been in any doubt about my intentions, I put him straight, telling him: 'Absolutely not! No way am I letting the team down and not seeing through the last shows to the end. We've had a brilliant time in this panto and I'm playing the Wicked Queen, so at least I don't have to smile!' I joked. Gallows humour has always got me and the rest of the family through the dark moments in life.

But while I may have been able to temporarily hide from my cancer and block out what was happening while up on that stage, there was one person from whom I couldn't hide how I was really feeling.

'I can pretend none of this is happening until we get home to Blackpool, but you cannot be in the wings,' I told Brian the next day. 'Promise me. If I see you standing there, I will cry because then it makes it real.'

Curtain down on the last show it was time to get my high heels and glad rags on and go out and have a good time at the after-show party.

I love a party and I had been looking forward to this one. Letting my hair down helped to take my mind off cancer and for a couple of hours I felt like me again, not Linda Hudson, cancer patient.

Arriving home in Blackpool on the Monday, reality hit me. I was booked into the Victoria Hospital's breast care unit in the middle of the first week in February 2006, where I met the Breast Care Nurse Specialist assigned to me.

She is called Sarah Middleton and she was brilliant – a real straight talker, which I love – and she has since gone on to become one of my great friends.

We went into the room and greeted the doctor. Brian was there holding my hand and Coleen also came in to support me, which I was glad for. Mr Rajon was my surgeon, and he took me behind the screen to examine me and went to me, 'Oh, yes', as he felt the lump.

I knew from the expression on his face that he wasn't going to turn around, and – like in the imaginary conversation I'd been having with myself – tell me, 'Not to worry, Mrs Hudson, we have all made a terrible mistake and the lump is benign.'

As I was dressing, he was checking again through all the file notes that had been sent across from Belfast before breaking the news to me.

'Mrs Hudson, I'd like you to have a mastectomy followed by chemo and radiotherapy.'

'Okay', I said, because what else could I have said at that moment? You don't take in what you are being told when worries are going around your head such as: am I going to die; am I going to lose my hair; they want to take my breast off; what's Brian feeling; how's Brian; and, of course, work ... what will happen with my work?

The reason I left it for so long was that I had been working in a stage production of *Blood Brothers*, playing Mrs Johnston. Then we went on to Belfast to do this fabulous pantomime from the end of November until the end of January. There is no sick pay in showbiz, you see, and if we don't work, we don't get paid, so

I just thought, 'I will get these shows over with, then I will go to the doctors and have this thing checked out.'

Anyway, I really should not have thought that way because I could have died. And I will say to anybody reading this that if you have a lump or bump that's not going away, DO NOT WAIT. Please go and see your GP and have it looked at. It could save your life.

When we finished speaking about my diagnosis, I cried. Then they took me into a lovely side room where people who have received bad news are taken. I sat there with Sarah, my new breast cancer nurse, as they made an appointment for my surgery. She said, 'Well, we could do the next week.' And I went, 'Woah, wait a minute, I need to get my head around all of this. I can't go into surgery yet.'

My head was still spinning from the impact of the diagnosis and I was in no position to make any serious life-altering decisions. Brian sensibly asked, 'Will it make a difference?' and she said, 'No, two weeks won't make a difference; just some people like to go in and get it done straight away.'

We made the appointment for 21 February, two days before my 47th birthday, and then headed back to our best friends Sue and Graham, with whom Brian and I had been living.

To quickly explain our living circumstances at this point, before the cancer diagnosis we'd moved out of our place in Blackpool and we were going to relocate down to London again because we loved the city and Brian's son Lloyd and daughter Sarah live there but at the time, with the tour happening, it seemed a silly time to buy somewhere in a rush, so we stayed with our friends.

It sounds funny to say it but when I got my first diagnosis over in Ireland, I was embarrassed to tell them, so they were unaware what I was going through.

When we got back to the house from the hospital, I went straight up to my bedroom to freshen up and change, Brian following in my wake.

I tried to look like I was busy picking things up and tidying, so I did not have the awkward conversation I had been avoiding since our return, but there was no stopping him.

'Lin, why aren't you telling Graham and Sue that you've been told you've got breast cancer?' he urged.

I snapped back, 'I don't know, because I'm embarrassed.'

'Why are you embarrassed?' he asked in exasperation.

I was not able to answer him and even after all this time I still do not truly know why. It's weird to feel embarrassed because you have got cancer, but it was a feeling that was there.

It's the look that people give you in those circumstances, which I know they mean well by. I hate pity and I didn't want people to be speaking to me, their heads sympathetically cocked to the side.

Later that evening, when we were all sat down at the table, Brian went, 'I've got something to tell you.'

I glared at him as if to say that is not your business to tell. Ignoring my furious look, he said: 'Lin's been diagnosed with breast cancer.'

They both went, 'Oh my God.'

By that point I was mad with Brian. Glowering at him I left the table and charged upstairs. My eyes pricked with tears as he came running after me.

I turned and shouted, 'That was not your business to tell them!'

He said, 'Lin, you're living with these people. They love you and I don't understand why you're embarrassed by it.'

'It doesn't matter what you don't understand,' I yelled back, 'it was my news to give.'

Looking back at those events from where I'm sat now in my life, I can see that Brian was absolutely right to do what he did because, after it was said in the open, the whole atmosphere in the house was different.

From then on in I could chat away to Sue about my cancer and the treatment instead of letting it become the proverbial elephant in the room.

On the other side it was a feeling of devastation and the more people you tell the more real it becomes. I remember I would just sit down to talk with somebody and in the middle of the conversation I would just start crying. I was so scared.

Looking back, the feelings of embarrassment I had suffered from were really partly terror and partly caused by having to talk about something that was very personal. The feeling of embarrassment stemmed from talking about my boobs to people and I was not comfortable with talking about changes that were happening to my body.

You see, we were not a family that was open when it came to personal matters. I never saw my mum and dad naked; we never ran around the house naked as children.

I think it's great that people these days are more open with their children and it's nothing for my nieces and nephews to see their mums and dads take a bath.

Now, all these years later, if somebody said to me, 'I'm just embarrassed by it', I would tell them I completely understand their embarrassment', I know the feeling, and I was embarrassed and upset about the changes like losing my hair too.

That is why I talk about it all now, because it can help somebody else who was once feeling the way I was. Somebody who may be thinking like I once did, 'Oh my God, I'm so embarrassed to tell my friends'. Or when they cannot understand that feeling of embarrassment, they know it's okay and not to worry. People say to me 'you're so open about it' or 'you have helped me through it', and I think, I will keep talking about these things because it all helps.

• • •

Once it was out about my cancer, my impending mastectomy was all I could think about.

Of course, everybody else had their own opinions about the treatment plan assigned for me, asking me questions like, 'why aren't they taking both your breasts away as isn't there a risk of cancer going to the other breast?'

I knew their messages were given with good intentions, but I started to worry that I was on the wrong course of action and, as the operation date grew closer, I started to feel jittery about it all.

I phoned Sarah, my breast cancer nurse, hoping she would help put my mind at rest.

After a couple of rings, Sarah picked up the phone and, typical me, I dived straight in by asking her if I should get a second opinion on the cancer.

'Oh, Linda,' she sighed with frustration. 'It was there! We could all see it' – as if to say, don't be ridiculous even thinking such a thing.

Hearing her reaction, I intuitively knew Sarah was my kind of person and exactly who I needed in my corner.

I did not want somebody sympathetically agreeing and pussyfooting around me. Lulling me into a false sense of security that everything was okay was not going to save my life. I needed honesty and I knew Sarah would never dress up the truth in front of me no matter how unpalatable.

I also asked her about the mastectomy and if I needed to have both breasts off, and she said, 'No, why would we take healthy tissue away, Linda? Why would we take something that's fine?'

She explained that as I did not have the BRCA gene, which is the gene for breast cancer, a double mastectomy would not be beneficial for me.

With that, I knew the treatment plan Blackpool Victoria Hospital had chosen for me was the best course of action and started to prepare.

My operation had been scheduled for the 21st, two days before my 47th birthday, and the hospital had requested that I come in for all the preliminary checks the night before.

But Brian called them up to ask if it would be okay for me to check in early on the morning of the op so I could spend a last evening with my family.

The hospital team were really understanding and lovely and said it would not be a problem if I came in that morning at 6.30am.

I have to say I cannot praise the NHS enough for the continuous care they have shown throughout this process. All the doctors and nurses who have cared for me over the years have been brilliant and, whenever there is a chance to clap for them, I am there.

You see, Brian and Coleen knew I would not have slept a wink, so they arranged a lovely meal out at one of my favourite restaurants for the four of us.

Brian got on brilliantly with Coleen's former husband Ray Fensome, so we spent quite a bit of time with Coleen in those days when she was married to Ray, and our nights out were always filled with laughter.

When we arrived at the restaurant, Coleen kept putting her head to one side and joked 'you're very brave, you're very brave', to which I kept saying, 'I'M NOT BRAVE, I have no choice!'

What else are you going to do in this situation, say no and die? Don't get me wrong, it's a lovely sentiment from people and I appreciate hearing it and would hate people to think that I was mocking, but I always find it funny how some folks react to friends and family with a life-threatening illness.

So often, when they walk towards you, the head cocks to one side and they tell you in sympathetic tones, 'You're very brave, you know'.

Brave or not, that night I tucked into my food with gusto as I knew I would be on hospital rations for the next few days, and after dinner we all headed to Coleen's house for a nightcap.

Walking up to the front door, I spotted a sign she had written, which made me laugh, it read, 'A Gathering for the Very Brave Linda Hudson'.

I thought, what on earth is going on here, only to walk through the front door and find all my family waiting to welcome me, which was lovely. It was just us, the family, together again, having fun and laughter to take my mind off the operation awaiting me, and I could not have asked for a better group of people to be related to.

We've always kind of dealt with stuff with humour. We know the moment to be sad or to be quiet or to be serious, but humour has got us through a lot of tough times, and that's how we are, you know. So if I had gotten in there and everybody was really serious, I would have gone, Oh, for God's sake, I'm losing my breasts, not my sense of humour. However, you have all lost your sense of humour, so get over it!

On the way back to Graham and Sue's house that night, I cried in the car because I love my family so much and they're gorgeous and I was scared – really scared – because I was frightened of dying and scared of the unknown.

I had spoken to Anne back then about it a lot because she was first diagnosed in 2000 and had made a full recovery. She would patiently answer my questions as I blurted out questions like what's chemo like and the other stuff you never normally would ask a cancer survivor unless you too were dealing with cancer. She was quite naturally brilliant and gave me a lot of comfort and guidance.

At that time, because there was no Covid, everybody was around the house with good wishes and it was very surreal, but I think I would hate it to be without laughter. I would hate it all to be serious because, as I say, there's plenty of time for being serious and being grown up if you like and having to sit there and not make jokes, so I wouldn't have wanted it any other way.

ANNE

The first time I had cancer I was given the all-clear after five years and I have lived every moment since in gratitude.

Life has been amazing between then and now but once you have had cancer whenever you get anything wrong with you, be it a sore toe or a bit of earache, your brain immediately goes on cancer-alert mode.

In 2000, when I first got told I had cancer, my life up to that point was by and large pretty good. I was happily married, we had two beautiful daughters, Amy and Alex, who were 12 and 18 at the time, and had no serious worries.

Over the years I'd already had several lumps removed from my breasts, which always turned out to be cysts.

Many women suffer with breast cysts throughout their lives and most of the time they are nothing to worry about, but you should always get anything you find investigated.

I regularly checked my breasts and when I would find a cyst, off I would pop to the doctor, who would examine me and then normally stick a needle in it to aspirate it and drain it away.

One morning I was doing my usual breast check – I cannot stress enough the importance of checking your breasts for changes – and I felt what I thought was to be another cyst.

I made my appointment with my local GP in Blackpool and they went through the normal assessment, said it was a cyst and got rid of it.

The GP then examined me again to check it was gone, but this time I could see from her reaction something was not quite right.

She said: 'Anne, I found another lump, which is very deep in your breast.'

'Are you sure?' I asked.

'Yes, I can feel it right here—' she put her hand back where the lump was buried '—I would like you to have it looked at as soon as possible and I'm going to send you for a mammogram at the breast unit to have it checked, just to be sure.'

I was not initially panicked at that point because I've had that many lumps removed and while she gave no indication as to whether it was serious or not, I didn't at that time think this might be or could be different; I just thought it's going to be assessed, I will have some examinations done and the mammogram, and I didn't think beyond that.

I got dressed again and went home as normal and I told my husband Brian, and my daughters, 'Oh, I've had that lump removed that I told you about, but the doctors found another one, so I've got to go and have a mammogram done and some tests done, and it will be fine, you know.'

The girls asked why I had to have another check and I told them it was normal procedure because this one was so deep in my breast that the doctor couldn't really tell what it was, and therefore that I was having the mammogram to determine it.

The hospital called me up and I was pencilled in for a mammogram. My husband came with me as we always did everything together.

Brian was six and a half years younger than me and he was only 19 when I met him, but he was an extraordinarily strong person, and he would always look on the positive side of life and tell you that you were going to be fine, which is exactly what I need.

And that is what he did that evening. He said, 'Anne, you're just going in to be assessed and it will be like all the other times.'

And we kind of just got on with our lives until we went into the hospital. I'd had mammograms before so I was not fazed by that and on that day, I told myself it was just another mammogram and I had a lump, but it was going to be assessed and it would be found to be benign.

Brian was thinking the same way as me because we had no reason to think differently really.

Although the doctor had sent me for a mammogram rather than just fixing it herself as she had the other lumps, my thinking was, because she can't get to the back of your breast that's why she sent me for a mammogram because she can't tell what it is.

You know, you kind of make yourself believe what you want to believe, I think. And that was our thoughts really, that she sent me for a mammogram because she could not get the lump out with the needle.

After the mammogram was done and dusted, Brian and I went home from the hospital like it was another ordinary day and forgot all about it while we waited for the results.

And then I had a phone call from the hospital.

The consultant's secretary told me they wanted me to go in and do a biopsy as soon as possible.

Things then suddenly got a bit more serious. I held the phone tight against my ear and asked her to repeat what she'd said because I was so shocked that I would need one.

She made an appointment for me and I thanked her and hung up the phone and went to tell Brian. I felt jittery and it was reflected in my voice as I said, 'Bri, that was the hospital telling me to, I think, to go in. They want to do a biopsy. Will you come with me?'

If Brian felt any worry about my medical situation, he did not show it as he jumped up and came over and put a reassuring arm around me and gave me a cuddle.

'Of course, I'm coming with you. It's going to be all right, please don't worry.'

And again, just hearing those words from him was immediately comforting, and I managed to stay calm until the day of my biopsy.

Brian came with me. He came with me for everything; no matter what it was he was so supportive, and he was – he is – just an amazing positive person, and an amazing husband, always offering words of encouragement.

Brian drove me in. We did not say much on the journey there, but he took my hand when we walked in – we always held hands – and was a solid comfortable presence.

'It's going to be all right, Anne,' he told me before we went in the room. The hospital gave permission for us to be in the room together while the biopsy was being carried out and that helped allay my fears, knowing he was there with me if I needed him at any point.

I'd never had a biopsy done before, and what they do is to insert a large needle into an area of concern to extract cells to test to check if they are malignant.

Now, you are probably wincing reading all the gory details but while it sounds nightmarish it was not a terrible, torturous pain. It was what I would describe as a bit sore and uncomfortable when the needle was going into the lump, but the needle was not sore going into the actual breast itself.

However, when I went to get off the bed afterwards it was a totally different matter.

The rush of pain that hit me was so sudden that it made me almost pass out.

Panicking, I said to the doctor and nurse, 'Oh, I … I don't feel well.'

Nothing like this had happened to me before; because I'd never had a biopsy before and didn't know what to expect, it was something of a shock, so I had to lie back down in the bed and Brian came and sat beside me and held my hand.

And then after about ten minutes I was okay. They checked me over and said I was okay to go home.

Looking down at my breast it was massively bruised and looked black, which kind of scared me, but the medical team weren't at all fazed by it, and said: 'that's nothing, there's nothing to worry about', and sent us home.

With the reaction to the biopsy being such a dramatic one, and my breast turning black and blue, by this time I was thinking, this is not going to be good, because I had plenty of cysts aspirated with a needle and nothing like that had happened before.

It started to play on my mind, and I kept thinking it over, and I think Brian probably felt the same, but he would never say that to me; he was always encouraging and saying that it was going to be fine.

This time while I tried to believe him, I started to think the worst and became anxious. That week felt the longest week of my life, waiting for the hospital to get in touch, and then we got the call to come back in for the results.

The night before receiving the results I felt nervous again because of that reaction to the biopsy. Half of me was thinking, what if it's not fine because I'm kind of a realist and think through all scenarios when I'm looking at something, so part of me was thinking it might be more than a cyst.

Brian was remaining optimistic, but I think as he had witnessed my breast turning black deep down he was feeling a little on edge and so neither of us could make ourselves think optimistically this is going to be 100 per cent okay and you'll be told it's nothing. As much as we may have liked to have thought that way, it just wasn't as easy this time.

The next morning was a bit of a blur; we got ready and headed over together to the hospital, trying not to dwell on what they were going to say.

The first clue was the Macmillan nurse who was standing with the consultant surgeon. I was then asked to take a seat.

Now, before I say what happens next, how about this for some nominative determinism. The consultant's name was Mr Pettit, would you believe? I almost got the giggles when I heard it.

But it was time to be serious and it got serious very quickly when Mr Pettit put his hand on my knee. Then I was focussing solely on him and not his name.

With his hand still on my knee and he said, 'Anne, I'm afraid it has come back as cancerous.'

The next few minutes were a blur as I tried to process what he'd just said. I think I replied 'okay' but I did not cry or freak out and neither did Brian.

We just kind of sat there for a couple of minutes in silence, having our own thoughts.

It felt surreal and like Linda, it almost felt like I was having an out-of-body experience in a way.

My brain was shutting down so I didn't have to think about what he'd just said; it felt like I had drifted off somewhere for a couple of minutes and this wasn't happening to me.

I'm not sure what pulled me back into the room, maybe my own survival fighting mechanism kicking in, because I looked right at the consultant and said, 'Okay, what happens next?'

Credit to Mr Pettit, who was an amazing surgeon and had a lovely way about him. He told me straight up, 'Well, you will have an operation to remove the lump and then you'd probably have chemotherapy and radiotherapy, but we'll decide after you've had your operation.'

And that was it really in a nutshell. I just thanked him, and he said, 'Well, you know, we'll be in touch about the time for your operation.'

With that, Brian and I walked out the hospital, hand in hand, in complete silence. We didn't say anything. We went through the motions of getting in the car and on the drive home neither of us spoke to one another; it was complete silence because I guess we were both lost in our own thoughts.

Also because I hadn't broken down or cried, I just hadn't even talked about it, I think Brian was doing what he thought I wanted him to do, which was to be there for me, and that if I wanted him to talk about it, I would let him know.

So, he was just reading me as he would never have wanted to have said or done the wrong thing.

I just didn't want to talk about it at that moment and the reason why was because I knew if I started talking about it, I probably would break down, and I still had to go home and tell our two daughters, so I had to just keep strong for them really.

When we got home, we both came in and I remember Alex, who was only 12, had one of her friends there after school.

They were looking at me expectantly with these big, bright smiles on their sweet faces, hoping that I was going to say, everything's fine.

However, I was a bit harsh really, and I wish I could go back and undo the way I told them because I just said to them bluntly,

'It's cancer, I'm afraid I've got cancer.'

They went, 'Oh, go away. You're joking.'

And I said, 'Girls, no, I'm not joking. I'm serious. I've got to have an operation.'

And I think because Brian and I were so calm about it in front of them, almost nonchalant when I think back to that day, they didn't break down.

I remember my eldest daughter telling me it wasn't until she walked around the park to discuss the news of my breast cancer with some of her aunts that she cried about it.

Brian and I were matter of fact the entire time with the children during my cancer, explaining that I would be having an operation to take the lump out and that I may have to have some medicine after that to get rid of the cancer.

I did try to make it all positive for them so that they didn't have to worry about it, but I do remember saying to them that I wanted them to know the truth, which that I was having this operation and it was going to be fine. I did not want to sugar coat it and lie to them about what was about to happen to me. I wanted them to know that there was a chance that it might not be fine. I didn't want them to go through it thinking, 'Oh, this is going to be great'. I wanted them to know that I had a life-threatening disease and that I might not come out the other end, and I wanted them to be prepared for that really.

This was to protect them, so they didn't think everything was going to be okay and I'd be home miraculously cured, and then all of a sudden, they'd have to be told it wasn't fine. You know, I wanted to prepare for the fact that it could turn around and that I could die from it. Now that's a hard thing for children to hear about their mum; looking back now I think I might have been a bit hard telling them that because Alex was only 12 and Amy was only 18, but I hoped I was being a sensible mother.

I didn't do this for any other reason than to help them really. That was my hope – that they would be prepared for all angles.

Then we approached the lumpectomy in the same way.

Brian and me were people then who take things in life as they come and deal with them when they arise.

I've had many traumatic things happen in my life, and he's always been there to hold my hand, guiding and supporting me through it.

Both the births of my daughters were terribly traumatic, and after those I had a gangrenous appendectomy and then cancer.

But throughout all my adversity Brian has always been there for me. He has been an absolute rock and support, and he's the one I've always gone to with anything I needed to talk about because I could tell him anything. If you spoke to anybody about Brian, they would say what a great guy he is and loved by his friends.

With this, obviously we talked about the lumpectomy and what was going to happen during the operation, how it would be afterwards, and we still didn't break down because we had to be strong for the two girls and the family.

There was a point where I did break down and cry and, when I did, Brian just held me in his arms and he was fabulous.

He was so strong, looking back, like how he knew that if I reacted badly to the chemo once I started, he was going to have to look after the girls while I was recovering.

A lot of men would have wobbled and crumbled straight away, yet Brian never once made any complaint, and I never heard him once moan, or groan about what he had to do.

He was and still is a wonderful father and I couldn't have had my children and career at the same time without him. I will always be grateful to him for that.

And it was a long drawn-out process – the chemo went on for six months and he had to not only look after my girls, but he also had to earn a living because he was the breadwinner. Later on, things did happen, which I talk about in depth further in the book, but initially I had no reasons to feel any concern about Brian at that point.

My main concern was the reaction of my children, how they were feeling and being supportive for them.

But Brian had to do all that for me because I was ill and I couldn't be there for them all in the way I wanted to be, so he had to be there for that. He was mum and dad and he had to be there for me as well.

When it came to my own breast operation, it's not pleasant by any means, but next to a mastectomy it's a much less invasive procedure and I feel very fortunate I didn't have to have my breasts removed.

You can preserve much of your breast with a lumpectomy including the sensation, and you recover quicker.

Both times I was in and out of hospital within a couple of days. The daunting part, next to making sure they have removed every bit of cancer there is, is the general anaesthetic to put you under, although some women opt for localised depending on the size of the lump you are having extracted.

And while rare, some women can be left disfigured by them if the lump was a significant size.

The first time I had my lumpectomy I was scared because I had never had one before, so the feeling of fear came from the unknown.

Brian took me into the hospital and my wonderful consultant came to speak to me and give the instructions to prepare me for the op.

The operation itself was a success. I was in surgery less than an hour, eating a few hours after I came around, and then back up and about the next day.

I'd already purchased soft bras with no underwiring in them for comfort for after the op and they were a godsend, as a lumpectomy does leave you with discomfort and some swelling, and the area was tender for several days.

I was also very fortunate to not have ended up with lymphoedema like poor Linda.

They gave me painkillers to dull the ache, and I rested at home for several days just pleased to know the cancerous lump was out of my body.

The surgeon did a good job too as the scar on my right breast was neat and I hadn't any long-lasting side effects.

Brian and my daughters really rallied around me, as did my sisters just as they do now. Having my daughters to think of as well and wanting their lives to go on as normally as possible was a great focus to bring me through what was a difficult time.

I did get through it and realised how lucky I was to have had that all-clear after five years although my world was to be turned upside down when Linda was diagnosed with breast cancer in 2006.

It was such a shock as it brought all those memories from my own battle flooding back and yet a completely different experience.

When somebody else has got cancer, you feel helpless and don't know what to do or say, even though you have been through it, because everybody's journey is different.

Even though I had a breast cancer operation, I didn't know what it was like to go through a mastectomy, which is an invasive operation far worse than a lumpectomy, and I didn't know what I could tell Linda. I felt quite helpless.

It brought back to me the memories of when I'd had cancer and how my family must have felt, not being able to do anything for me.

I didn't like to talk about my cancer to people – even now I struggle talking about it – so I dealt with it in my own way and if I wanted to talk or ask a question I would.

But when it came to Linda and then Bernie, how you approach it, or your opinions on it, goes flying out the window. You are there for them 100 per cent because they are your sisters who need your love and your support.

You stop thinking about yourself and you think only about them and what they need and are there for them all the way.

Partly I think that is because we are a big family so we've always been there for each other and rally around each other no matter what's happening.

I know Maureen thinks about me before herself and the same for Denise, who is looking after Linda; she will be thinking of Linda first before she thinks about what she wants to do. It feels like it is something innate in each of us in the family to come together at times of need and peril and be there for each other. I look around and see each of us in our family are very lucky to have this amazing Nolan support network to call on.

It also helps that geographically apart from Coleen – who is living in Cheshire, which is an hour away – we are all located near one another in Blackpool and subsequently we see each other at least four times a week when there are no Covid restrictions. I can walk to Lin and Denise's in ten minutes. I don't think I would have been able to have got through this big fight with cancer without them.

But I also could not have got through what I have been through without the love and support of my two daughters.

Looking back on that time and what my daughters went through the first time with me at such a tender age, they were even more amazing this time because they were now adults with children of their own and understood about life more.

My daughters have been through a great deal, as well as my sisters and brothers, but they are great at putting me straight.

If I ever phone up going, 'Oh God, I have to have chemotherapy again. I'm not having it', they'll go, 'Yes, you are having it, Mother.'

They know exactly what to say to me and they don't even discuss the fact that I'm insisting on not having it and just ignore me and tell me off.

The girls have such belief in me and if I'm ever having a wobble, both of them have said to me at different times, 'Mum, you've been through so much and you have to go through it again.

'You fought it successfully before and you will fight it again and if it comes back, we are all there and we will get through it again.'

They're so strong; Brian and I must have done something right along the way.

My sisters and my girls are very close; I'm sure they've probably talked to their aunties and broken down. In fact, I know they have. I asked them, 'You know, how have you been doing'. And they told me they've cried a lot and been angry, but when they talk to me, they never cry and they don't even sound like they're down about it. They always sound positive about it and I know that's to protect me; they always try to make me feel positive as well.

Their reaction is always, 'No, Mum, you'll get through it.' Or, they'll tell me, 'Look what you've been through already.' That's the kind of attitude they have – truly amazing.

And the other thing I love about how they've handled this whole experience for the last two decades is that they've passed it down to their children, my grandchildren, who also have that kind of positive gung-ho attitude.

I lost all my hair but my granddaughter is so blasé and matter of fact about it and does not care if I have hair or not.

I was saying to them one day, 'Oh God, I'm so fed up with feeling ill. I just want to feel well again.'

And my 12-year-old grandson said to me, 'You will feel well again, Gran, it's just taking a bit of time, that's all.'

12 and speaking with such maturity and sensitivity; I'm constantly amazed by them all. And it's credit to the girls who have told the grandchildren how it is and stopped them from being fearful.

Knowing they believe I will get through this again inspires me to keep on going.

I suppose having come through what I did the first time is what is so surreal about all of this.

It was so quick and sudden after being on that fantastic cruise for two weeks, then watching the amazing series on TV and next thing somebody tells you have cancer and will need chemotherapy.

Like the spread of the Covid pandemic it all happened so fast I could not process it.

One minute I'm on this cruise and the next I'm having needles pumped in me with chemotherapy.

It was horrendous and all our lives and world just changed, not just for me and Linda, but for all of us, because Denise was looking after Linda, so her life changed too. She has somebody else in the house, 24 hours a day, seven days a week, which she's not used to.

Maureen actually moved out of her house into my home, which was life-changing for her as well, as she had times when she couldn't go and see her grandchildren, because of Covid and nursing me meant she had to shield so as to not catch it and pass it on. The world had turned upside down for us all and I wondered when would this nightmare end?

CHAPTER 3

REMOVAL

LINDA

The first thing I did after the effects of the anaesthetic had worn off was lift up the bedsheet and check what it looked like.

'Oh, they've taken it!' I exclaimed to myself like there had been any doubt that they would leave my breast attached to me.

Where my left breast had once resided were bandages and padding so I wasn't able to see what it actually looked like, but there was no mistaking it: my skilled surgeon had done his work well … my breast was most definitely gone.

Pulling the sheet back up to my chin, I lay there staring up at the ceiling, just hoping that – with my left breast whipped off and in some hospital waste bin – all of the cancer had also gone on its merry way into the disposal unit.

However, if there were any stray cells lurking in my body, the chemo and radiotherapy would hoover them all up and zap them for me.

Surprisingly, for an amputation operation, I initially wasn't in the sort of searing pain I had been dreading – that may have been the morphine – and Brian was also there with me, which helped to take my mind off the fact I was now missing one of my boobs.

The family did come to visit in the evening, but they looked dismayed when they first saw me sitting up in bed with a smile on my face.

'Oh, I'm so disappointed,' Coleen jokingly said.

'So am I!' echoed Maureen.

Charming!

They told me, 'It's because we expected you to be delirious and lying swathed in bandages.'

'Oh, well, you know, I'm just very brave,' I replied, laughing, as they made themselves at home around my bedside.

I always love seeing my sisters and brothers on any day of the week but that day I especially did. When you have cannulas coming out of you and part of you is taped up like an Egyptian mummy and you're trying to not feel sorry for yourself, there is nothing better to snap you out your pity party for one than the company of your family.

Having them there gave me the sense of normality I had been craving. Our conversations often have an element of humour to them and when you are lying there, bruised, with a drain line sticking out your body, having your family around to tease and have a joke with is the best medicine there is, because it's a reminder of who you used to be before cancer.

It was funny what Coleen said and it made me laugh out loud. She has always got a funny line, has Coleen, she always cracks me up.

I know that they were scared coming to see me, and that me being wrapped in bandages is exactly what they had been dreading. The fact that I was sitting up wide awake, talking to them when they got there, meant the relief was palpable for Coleen, when she said, 'Oh my God, you're not swathed in bandages'.

She was thrilled really; when she said it like, I am *so* disappointed, it's because that's what we do to deflect from a situation. Humour is a massive thing in our lives and in our family, with everything that we deal with.

We will and can deal with stuff in a serious way, but then humour always creeps in. I can sit down and have a serious conversation with them when a serious conversation is needed but I think that to try and make light of things is sometimes the best way. They know I had a serious major operation, they know I had a mastectomy and I've got cancer, so I can only imagine what they were going through, waiting to come and see me. And then when they did see me, I think the relief was clear in their joking.

As the girls sat around my bed, nattering and eating all the chocolates they had brought to me, I felt impressed at myself for how I was handling the situation so remarkably well.

Here I am, I thought, being all jolly and upbeat as though having mastectomies and dealing with breast cancer was all in a day's work for me.

But the next morning when on my own my bravado deflated faster than a popped balloon after one of the nurses came in to speak to me.

I eyed her suspiciously, wondering what she wanted as she hovered by my bed.

'I'm here to dress your wound; how do you feel?' she politely asked.

'Fine,' I replied, while clutching my gown protectively to my chest.

'What I mean,' she said, 'is that some women don't like to see it, some women do, so I'm just going to re-dress it and need to know if you're ready to see it before I start?'

Then reality kicked in and I knew I could not yet face looking at the wound.

I told her, 'No, I'm not ready yet,' and the nurse nodded. I turned my head away to the side and I recall she was very gentle with me, slowly and carefully changing the dressing to make sure I didn't see anything.

But it's a shock because a part of who you are is not there – part of being a woman – and I felt disfigured. I haven't had reconstructive surgery yet because the hospital doing the mastectomy didn't offer it and I had to wait until I was assigned a spot at Wythenshawe Hospital, Manchester. Also, as well as physically, you have to be mentally strong enough to go through a major operation like reconstruction.

Bernie was there one day when the nurse was changing the dressing and she said, 'Oh you should look, Linda, it's unbelievable,' and I did then.

It's a shock when you first see it. It's flat and there's a scar across the centre where your boob should be, but the surgery was unbelievable because it was so neat.

Emotionally it didn't hit me until later on and that is the truth.

During that first cancer battle, as well as having the backing of my sisters and brothers, I do not know what I would have done without the love and support of my husband Brian. He was amazing, my rock, always caring and looking out for me.

In the following days, as I lay in the hospital bed, Brian went and got permission from the ward and spent ages Blu-tacking 'get well soon' and birthday cards onto the walls to cheer up the place and give me a reminder of home.

He was always thoughtful like that.

Despite everybody's best efforts to take my mind off the enormity of what I was going through, when I woke up in hospital that week on the morning of my 47th birthday, I had a bad case of the birthday blues.

The shock of having my breast removed hit home and I was aware that I had a big journey ahead of me to fight this disease. Other thoughts crept into my mind like what's it going to be like in the bedroom?

I was so down. All I wanted to do was hide from the world under the covers. And then Brian phoned me to sing me 'Happy Birthday', and all my emotions got the better of me and I sobbed down the phone to him.

The poor man must have thought it was his singing that set me off crying.

Can you believe it, but he got a speeding ticket that day because he was that worried about me from the way I sounded that as soon as he hung up the phone he jumped in the car and drove over to the hospital like he was Lewis Hamilton.

The sight of him arriving in the ward carrying a bunch of balloons and flowers lifted my spirits no end, and my sisters and brothers followed him bringing me a selection of lovely tops to wear and special post-surgery bras to hold a prosthesis – a foam spongy thing to protect your scar while it heals – which I had to wear until I was to be given my breast reconstruction operation.

Some women have theirs done straight away but talking to Sarah my breast cancer care nurse it was felt I was not mentally ready as well as physically ready and I did not end up having it for another 18 months or so for reasons that will become clear through the rest of this story.

Spending your birthday in hospital sucks but the love in the room that day was incredible and made up for being sick and stuck in a bed.

My other sister Denise was working on a cruise liner with her fiancé Tom, and they also phoned me on the morning of my birthday from Vietnam.

Denise never misses a birthday – never – and that made me cry because it was thoughtful of her and it must have been a nightmare trying to get through to the hospital.

To cap it all off, the nurses came in with a lovely birthday cake to wish me many happy returns. Looking back on it now, as birthdays go it was pretty special, and what my family did really helped lift my spirits.

Then, with all the fuss and business of the day over, it was time to sleep.

As soon as my eyes closed – even though Brian was not there beside me – I was out for the count. My body and my mind needed it, I guess.

After a week inside the hospital I was starting to get cabin fever. Fortunately, my superstar surgeon said he was pleased with my progress and said it was fine for me to carry on my healing at home while preparing to start my chemotherapy.

My breast care nurse Sarah was always fabulous company. She would come to see me in the hospital each day and had this unique way of announcing her presence, which was to pop her hand around the door, waving a tissue.

Let me assure you, Sarah was not practising her version of the Royal Wave on me, nor was she eccentric.

You see, every time I saw her all I could do was bawl my eyes out, so to make light of my tears, Sarah would always bring a hanky and do this jokey entrance.

'It's just as well I'm hard and I'm not getting upset by this,' I told her, my tears quickly turning to laughter, and she would fire back, 'I'm your reality check'. She was a breath of fresh air.

Sarah was quite simply brilliant. Her no-nonsense and straight-talking attitude got me through those tough moments as she did not mind answering the difficult questions that Brian would never dare to ask in front of me: questions such as what is Linda's prognosis or what has worked or not worked?

When I asked if the surgery had got rid of the cancer for good, Sarah did not dress things up by which I mean give me false hope. She answered truthfully: 'We don't know yet because we have to get all the results back. But they have got everything out and they've taken out eleven infected lymph nodes. The lump was the size of a small courgette.'

'Well, we won't be eating ratatouille again!' I exclaimed, at which she laughed her head off.

'Seriously though, Linda, you are so lucky. Another couple of weeks even …' she replied, reminding me of how close I had left it.

She wasn't implying I would have dropped dead but prior to the surgery they didn't have all the information that it had spread to the lymph nodes and how bad they were.

Agreeing with her, I said: 'I know, and I've been an idiot.'

In your dream world you think you have life and everything under control, when more often than not, you don't. That's why I say to people: please do not be like me. If I had gone sooner to the doctor it may have just been a lumpectomy like Anne's was; she was in and out of hospital in a day.

I then had two weeks' recuperation time back home before my chemotherapy started, and I had to face up to life without my left breast for the next 18 months until I was able to have reconstruction.

Marilyn Monroe said she wore nothing to bed except a few drops of Chanel No 5, but after my mastectomy all that went out the window for me. I didn't want to be naked in front of Brian as I couldn't bear him to see my scar, or touch it, but I didn't have my own nightwear, so I started wearing Brian's T-shirts to bed so that I kept the scar covered.

It was such a traumatic thing for us as a couple dealing with the effects of my mastectomy. Brian was going to me, 'I hope you don't think that's what we're all about, that all I loved you for is your boobs and your hair and all of that.'

My breasts had been such a part of my identity and I was known in the band as the one with the big boobs and blonde hair.

On seeing the hurt and upset on his face, I softened and said, 'Darling, I know that, but this is not about you.'

'Linda,' he continued, 'I don't mind.'

'Yeah, I know that Brian, but the difference is I do mind, and it's not about you, I swear to God. It's about me and how I feel, and I have to get through this, so please give me time,' I pleaded, 'and bear with me.' Because *to me* it was ugly, and I missed my breast.

So, despite Brian's protestations, I carried on wearing a T-shirt in bed every night for the next couple of months.

Every time I had a shower and saw the scar it reminded me of having cancer. I hated looking at it and seeing a flat space on my chest wall where my breast used to be, so I would cover up wherever possible to avoid being reminded that I had cancer.

Another annoying side effect while I was waiting for my breast reconstruction was wearing these bras with the prosthesis in them.

Trying to get it on and off was a struggle as I had developed lymphoedema in my left arm, which plagues me to this day. Lymphoedema is when one or both arms or legs swell up. It's caused by removal of or damage to the lymph nodes as part of your cancer treatment. What happens is that there's a blockage in your lymphatic system and this blockage prevents lymph fluid from draining well. The fluid then builds up because it can't escape and that leads to the swelling and your limbs can really widen, making it a problem with clothes.

It's the reason why I always wear loose tops for the ease of getting them over my arm. There are treatments that help to reduce it and I've tried them, but you must work at it, so I have learned how to live with it.

But on that day, it became a real problem. Anne was coming over to meet me and we were going out for lunch, but I could not get the bra's back strap to fasten because of the swelling and I was having real trouble.

Anne arrived and wondered what was taking me so long. I explained and she said to me, 'Do you want me to do it?'

I asked if she was sure she wanted to help because she might not want to see the mastectomy, but Anne was having none of it and told me not to be ridiculous and came up and got it straight on and fastened it.

To help deal with my fears and regain my body confidence I realised I needed some professional guidance, so I started speaking to a consultant clinical psychologist who specialises in cancer, called Dr Jean Brigg – I still see her now. I started seeing her on the advice of Sarah because I thought I was going mad. I started the menopause aged 47. It happened after my first chemo. I was getting menopausal mood swings with Brian and thought this is mental.

Along with Sarah, and the wonderful medical team, Dr Jean was another great help in my cancer journey, giving me new ways of coping and coming to terms with the massive physical and psychological change to my body. She was fabulous and brilliant with all of that.

I didn't know what to do at first as I had never had any therapy or counselling before and it was all new to me, but I gave it a go and within ten minutes of being in there I was breaking my heart crying. It was a release to speak to somebody that was not family, so I did not have to worry about upsetting them about how I felt about everything. She explained to me about the menopause and I told her a couple of incidents I will discuss later in the book. She said *your way* to deal with it, Linda is to sleep through it and that is amazing – that your way is to step away from the situation. I think our relationship developed from there.

That is not a tip – she was talking to me about how I had reacted to being plunged into a menopause and that rather than taking loads of medication for the hot flushes my method that worked for my symptoms was to sleep.

I would see her once every three weeks at that time and we spoke about cancer and how it was difficult for me to undress in front of Brian, and I told her one afternoon about my struggle with sleeping naked next to Brian and how I had resorted to wearing his old T-shirts to bed, but not being able to lie there bare skinned in bed next to him did not feel the same and I was missing our intimacy.

She said to me, 'Stop wearing his T-shirts and just buy some lovely new T-shirts, Linda, or a nice camisole top. Brian is fabulous in what he said and he's not pressuring you', and so that is what I did.

It was difficult for me and it was difficult for Brian at that time because when you are in it and the one dealing with cancer you do not realise you are being unreasonable at times and the other person is also finding their way through it and learning how to adjust to all the changes.

Then I just remember one day when I was getting changed, I had a feeling I was ready to show Brian my scar.

Until this point if Brian was to walk in the room when I was getting dressed, I would turn my back on him and shy away, but this time I decided I was ready to face my fears.

He came into the bedroom as I was putting on my clothes and I did not move. I faced him defiantly with my chest out and he spoke to me like normal, never flinching or staring in disgust as I once had feared, and then he went back out.

'I did it!' I told myself. This was a big step forward for me. Then a moment later he came back in and he gave me a hug and went, 'I love you'. He was amazing, and I told him again how I had only been wearing a T-shirt at night because I felt ugly, and he held me and said, 'I know'.

With these things you have to do it your own way in your own time; you cannot be cajoled or pushed, and to be fair to Brian he did not ever ask like some selfish blokes probably would, 'Do you not want to sleep with me or something?'

He was sensitive and understanding.

• • •

As I prepared for chemotherapy, arranged by my consultant clinical oncologist Dr Shabbir Susnerwala, I still had not made up my mind if I wanted to have Brian there with me during treatment but had not told him how I was feeling.

He took me to the hospital. I was quiet in the car as I contemplated if it was right for Brian to come in with me.

The reason I worried was simply because I did not know what chemo was going to be like. You hear horror stories about it, and I had no idea what to expect; whether I would be sat there vomiting or with my hair falling out in clumps. I had no idea, and I didn't want to inflict any more distress or heartache on Brian; he had been through too much as it was.

We parked up and, taking my hand, he walked me into the hospital. As we reached the entrance, I stopped suddenly.

Brian put his arm around me and gently kissed me. 'Come on, Lin, we'll be fine,' he said, thinking I was scared to go in.

I turned to face him, stopping him in his tracks.

'Brian, you know I love you more than life, but I think I'm braver if you're not there,' I said. 'I think if you're there I will fall into a heap and feel sorry for myself, but if you're not there I'll be brave and have to get on with it.'

Brian nodded and gave me a huge hug. He told me to phone him and he would come back to pick me up.

And with that I stepped out on my own and into the lion's den.

Having now been through chemotherapy multiple times, when I look back, the first session I ever had was not too uncomfortable as things went and, surprisingly, I felt okay.

Brian collected me and I felt a little tired but nothing as bad as what I had been expecting. In fact, I was ravenous and tucked into dinner with gusto when I got home.

But my chemo reprieve was short-lived. Later that night in bed all hell erupted, or shall I say *I* erupted – 22 times, in fact.

I vomited that many times through the night and into the next day that I thought I was going to bring up an organ. It was horrendous. I felt like it would never stop and just when I thought there was nothing more to come up, I would be sick again.

Brian was worried and, in between throwing up, I cried, 'If chemo is always going to be like this, I'm not doing it!'

When I was coming out of the bathroom, having hurled my guts up for the umpteenth time, I passed my friend Sue on the landing.

It was about half past six in the morning and she was getting ready for work. Her expression on seeing me was one of horror and she told me she thought I was dying so grey was my complexion.

Brian held similar fears, and taking one look at my pasty pallor, said: 'I'm calling the doctor, Lin; something's not right here.'

He phoned the brilliant team on the oncology ward who told him it was nothing relating to my chemotherapy but was gastroenteritis, which I must have picked up while on the ward.

Well, they sent over this special anti-sickness tablet to the house and it was a little bit of heaven because the minute I took the tablet I stopped vomiting. Talk about going from meh to yay in a few minutes. I felt human again and spent the rest of the day napping to make up for all my lost hours of sleep.

Chemo did other horrible things to my body, and it makes me feel ill thinking about that time and experience. Once every three weeks I would lose my taste buds completely. This would last for up to two and a half weeks and I had no taste for anything.

It was also a dangerous side effect because water tasted weird and disgusting – sometimes it would taste of salt, other times it would taste of metal – so I had no desire to drink it and ended up severely dehydrated and had to be put on a drip.

Now, being from Ireland, we Irish do like a nice cup of builder's tea, but I could not even drink that. The only liquid that broke through my palate was raspberry tea and so there I would be chugging back on cups of raspberry tea like it was going out of fashion.

Then for the next two or three days my taste buds would temporarily recover, so in that short window Brian would go mad getting me everything I loved to eat, or we'd go out for dinner or lunch and I'd gorge at my favourite restaurants knowing that for the next two and half weeks I would be back to not being able to eat anything.

The other ball ache was quite literally that – the aches. Some days I would wake up and every part of me would be racked with pain like the muscle and joint aches you have with a terrible bout of flu.

Thankfully, I did not have to work at that point, so I used to just stay in bed or, if the weather was nice, I would venture outside to get some fresh air and try to take a little walk.

It sounds vain that when I was facing a possible death sentence the thing I was worried the most about during the whole thing was losing my hair.

For me, the cold cap was a brilliant godsend and if you're going through chemo, I say give it a try. It is uncomfortable initially and a bit of a shock, but after about five minutes you adjust to the sensation and forget you're wearing it.

When you're fighting cancer, your body, skin and hair sadly cannot stay in its normal great condition, no matter how much you take measures to combat it.

Many medications do cause side effects, including thinning hair, and while I never had any actual bald patches the first time I had chemotherapy, sadly loads of my hair did fall out. The hair that was left turned steel grey and from a distance it looked like those Brillo pads you use to clean your greasy pans, as it was quite curly, but when you touched it, it was soft like baby hair.

To protect my straggly lank locks, I would wear what hair I had remaining up in a clip in the back of my head, but I did not care about its poor condition because I was so pleased just to have some hair left and knew it would thicken up once the chemo was over.

During my chemo I went back to work because I had to. In the world of entertainment, the bills do not get paid if you're not working.

Brian and I worked together and there was no money coming in from elsewhere because he had been having treatment for skin cancer – he was diagnosed before me in 2005 – so I had no choice but to carry on with the *Blood Brothers* tour.

There is no sick pay to cover you, and while we had life insurance, we had not taken out critical care cover, which would have afforded us the chance to take time off. My advice to anybody, whatever their profession or age, is to have critical care if they can afford it.

It is an expensive premium to pay but it is amazing if you are suffering from a long-term illness as it stops you worrying about money, and you can just concentrate on getting well.

A sick friend got £150,000 through her critical care and thank God my sister Bernie had taken out her own policy before she got cancer. She was awarded a hefty insurance payout, so she was spared worrying about working or where to get the money to pay the bills during her treatment.

Some have asked if being at work during that time was cathartic and helped to cause a distraction from cancer. Well, the answer to that is absolutely not. If I had a choice I would not have gone back until I had finished all my treatment, because it was so hard doing both.

I also suppose because Mum and Dad were singers, and performing was our life, we were taught from an early age from them that no matter what, the show must always go on.

When I was performing in the West End, I did not have the full company for the entirety of my eight-week stint because there is always somebody off with a migraine or sickness and diarrhoea or they've stubbed their toe or broken a nail.

I used to joke to Brian, 'One day I will have the whole company to work with.'

Well, that never happened. Apparently in the West End you have to take time off if you are ill and your understudy will step in to cover, but to me it was hilarious because as far as we were concerned as Nolans, unless you were a stretcher case you went on and did the show and then you went back to your sick bed.

The girl who understudied me used to say, 'Oh, I hate working with the Nolans because they're never off' and she never got her chance to play the part.

My life was suddenly turned into a military operation, such was the level of detailed planning required for me to undergo chemotherapy and still work full-time as an actress on the stage.

We had a system to make it work around my treatment schedule. If we opened the show for press night on the Monday, Brian and me would pack up, travel to the venue on the Sunday night, perform Monday and Tuesday night and then Brian would drive me back to Blackpool on the Wednesday. Then on Thursday I'd have my bloods taken ahead of undergoing chemo on the Friday. After chemo on the Friday we would then reload the car and drive back for the two shows on the Saturday. It was the hardest thing I think I have ever done, and I was exhausted.

To top it all off my eyelashes fell out and my eyebrows disappeared, so there was that to contend with, and then I also began suffering from terrible hot flushes that could come out of nowhere and leave me red and profusely sweating.

Those adverse reactions really did take their toll on me and I remember one afternoon in my dressing room, while getting ready for a performance, trying to draw eyebrows on only for them to melt off and run down my face, I turned to Brian and shouted, 'I can't do this anymore!'

I really had come to the end of my tether, but the cast were amazing with my illness and gave me a lot of support. Every time we stopped during rehearsals, they would be running up with a chair for me to sit on or somebody would bring me a fan to cool off with or a drink.

The director also let me do it wearing my slippers instead of shoes, because one of the side effects of Herceptin and chemo combined was that I got great big blisters on the soles of my feet, causing such terrible pains that I couldn't walk.

This stage family I worked with did become a family to me in the coming months of the tour. The actors playing my eight children would call me Mam, not Linda. If you played Mrs Johnstone in that show, you are mother to them forever. They call me Mam on birthday messages, and I call them my showbiz children. It's a lovely tradition and link to the tour, which I'm glad has continued until this day.

You may wonder if all the stress and exhaustion affected my performance? Well, I did get a dodgy review one night in Bath. The critic said I did not reach the high notes!

Normally I would not take such reviews to heart, but I remember that comment frustrated me because I knew it had nothing to do with my musicality and technique. I'd had chemo at 9am then travelled all the way to Bath and did the show that night and yes, I did not hit that high note, but I was there, I showed up.

Of course, you can't phone up the newspaper and tell them, 'Do you know what I'm going through? I'd like to see you try singing after having chemotherapy', because then it sounds like you can't take a bad critique.

However, I did throw the paper in the bin and shouted, 'Arseholes!' Made me feel much better.

CHAPTER 4

CHEMO WARFARE

LINDA

People have bad days during chemo treatment, and it can happen at any time: some people react badly the next day: other people might be okay initially and then have a bad day in the middle of the week.

My bad day usually hit me on day six or seven after chemo and I would wake up feeling like I was coming down with the flu. I would sit on the edge of the bed, feeling hot with terrible aching muscles, and Brian would go, 'You all right, babe?', and I would tell him that it was my sixth or seventh day.

Angel that he was, he would get up and make me a cup of tea and, my body wiped out, I would sleep off the effects for the rest of the day.

Eventually the chemotherapy ended and then it was on to radiotherapy. I had this daily Monday to Friday for four weeks in Preston, not Blackpool.

For those who have been lucky enough to never have had radiotherapy, in your first appointment they have to prep your body for the radiation by tattooing it.

A machine tattoos these tiny spots on your body where the radiotherapy is aimed at and I've got tiny tattoos around my boob and under my arm.

And so, if I'm ever asked if I have a tattoo, I tell them 'Yes, I do', and it's always fun to see the surprised look on their faces. They ask, 'Oh, what's it like?' And when I say it looks like a black-head, they do not know whether I'm joking with them or not.

This tattooing part is quite a long appointment because they must have everything exact and accurate to what the radiographer and consultant want, and there cannot be any room for error.

But once the markings are permanently etched onto your skin, the actual radiotherapy process moves fast. Put it this way: I would arrive in the morning at ten to ten on the dot, have a cup of tea, then the team would call me through, blast me with radiation and I would be back in the car in little more than 30 minutes.

During chemotherapy I held it together but when I underwent radiotherapy, it was the only time I would feel myself become emotional. The staff would lie me on the bed and walk out the room as the machine zapped me and during those moments is when I would let myself feel sad and have a big tear come down my face.

The side effects from radiotherapy were thankfully minimal. The worst I suffered was a little skin infection from a burn, and tiredness is also a common ailment, but next to chemotherapy, radiotherapy was a breeze.

Of course, I used to the tiredness card to my advantage when hanging out with my family and I wanted the sofa all to myself.

Visiting my nieces and nephews when I was first suffering from cancer, I would walk in a room and they would all jump up and say, 'Sit down, Aunty Linda', fussing after me like I was the Queen of Sheba. But months down the line the novelty of me being an invalid had worn thin and I was no longer given the special treatment.

'Aunty Linda is pretending to be sick again!' shouted the kids when I waved my cancer card* in front of them in a bid to make one of them feel sorry for me and give me the sofa.

(*My friend in Wales did really make me a 'cancer card'. It looks like a credit card, but it has got the pink ribbon on it and if queuing for a restaurant the girls would say, 'get the cancer card out, Linda!')

Kids are great for helping to make things feel normal and when you have cancer you learn to never take normal for granted again and are grateful for the mundane, for family life with all its ups and downs. You cannot put a price on that feeling of just having everyday problems to worry about until you have terminal illness.

The times I have wished I could just close my front door, lie on my sofa snuggled under the duvet, switch off my phone, pour a glass of wine and say to everybody to go away, but when you are battling cancer you can't do that because your whole life is surrounded by appointments. Be it blood checks one day or scans the next, cancer infiltrates every area of your life.

Living with cancer is like living with a caged tiger. It's completely unpredictable and can rise up and attack at any moment, so you are always in defence mode.

I had to deal with all the lovely side effects of chemo while also going through the menopause.

I didn't know this at the start, so spent ages worrying why one moment I would be feeling fine, having gone out with friends for a meal, enjoying the food, the ambience, and then, boom, out of nowhere there's a switch and the smell of food would make my stomach heave, leaving me suddenly fearing I would be sick at the table.

Or I would be out with friends having a light conversation and then from out of nowhere I would start crying.

My husband was a bloody saint to put up with my erratic mood swings during chemo. I could be laughing and joking one moment and then in high dudgeon the next.

He was amazing even when I was at my most unreasonable and irritable, snapping at him for no reason. I remember one Sunday while I was undergoing chemo, when I had developed a little bit of an appetite, we decided to take advantage of my taste buds returning and make a Sunday roast dinner.

There were a few things missing from our fridge and store cupboard, so I wrote a shopping list and on it was Aunt Bessie's Yorkshire puddings and various other things we needed for the roast, and I told him I would love some orange ice lollies.

The request for ice lollies is because when my taste buds would go awry with chemo, one of the few things I could stomach were Orange Maids orange-flavoured ice lollies, which are delicious.

Brian took the list and went off on his shopping mission while I attempted to clean up the kitchen and fridge in preparation for cooking.

An hour or so later, Brian returned, brandishing shopping bags triumphantly and looking rather pleased with himself.

He chatted away merrily, and his bizarre jolly tone immediately got on my nerves.

'There wasn't any Aunt Bessie's so I've got you some flour to make Yorkshire puddings with and there wasn't any ice lollies but … I've got you some orange jelly,' he announced gleefully, waving the box around in his hand like it was a cheque for a million pounds.

I looked at him and said, 'Orange jelly?'

'Yeah, well, you know how your taste buds are funny and you like the orange ice lollies and I like orange jelly, so I thought I'd get some for dessert afterwards …' he prattled on, trying to placate me.

'Orange fucking jelly! Who buys fucking orange jelly? I asked for Aunt Bessie's Yorkshire puddings!' I yelled, not recognising this shrill-sounding harridan I had seemingly turned into overnight.

Continuing with this orange-themed tirade of mine, poor Brian said 'Lin, I'm walking away from this' and as he did I launched the flour at him!

It missed Brian but burst halfway and covered the apartment in flour like a snowstorm.

I stormed past him and upstairs to bed where I slept for six hours solid.

I woke up later feeling my old cheery self and went to find Brian sat on the sofa, watching the television. I immediately went over and gave him a loving kiss.

'Brian, I'm so sorry. I don't actually know what happened before and I didn't mean to get so upset over Aunt Bessie's Yorkshires and a packet of jelly. Please can we forget about it?'

Brian was always understanding and like a good sport said, after my apology, 'I know it wasn't you, don't worry'. He knew I was not being myself and we ended up laughing about it.

He was always thinking of me and making sure I had everything I needed and that I was taken care of.

When my hair was thinning due to the chemo treatment, I'd go upstairs to bed, with no idea that Brian would get out the gaffer tape and dustpan and brush to pick up all my blonde hairs lying around so I didn't see that my hair was falling out.

Little did I know then that soon I would be the one helping Brian into hospital.

CHAPTER 5

LIFE OF BRIAN

Our husbands – both called Brian – played a mammoth and integral part in our lives and we cannot write this diary about our cancer journey without mentioning them.

Our marriages ended for different reasons – one of us is divorced; the other is widowed – but on the whole they were very happy, and we are each grateful to our respective other halves for the love and help they gave us during our first battles with cancer. They will forever be a part of our life story.

LINDA

My husband Brian died in 2007, on 21 September. There was a time I could not bear to talk about what I'm now going to say because of the extreme pain it caused me.

Brian drank a lot, and it took me a long time to say it after he died, but he was a functioning alcoholic.

Some mornings I would walk into the kitchen and find him drinking out a glass and he would say he had just been drinking Diet Coke. When he'd go to the loo I would smell the glass; he'd come in and I'd go, there's whisky in there and he'd go no, no, it's just last night's glass, and I'd go, yeah, well, do me a favour and get a fresh one, knowing it wasn't last night's glass.

So why did I not make Brian seek help?

Part of it maybe was denial. Brian had drunk all his life; he'd been in bands and – I'm not making an excuse for it – but there's a drinking culture in that world.

I think the reason I never initially said he was an alcoholic is not just a simple case of denial or putting my head in the sand, but because my image then of an alcoholic is a person falling over drunk and lying in the gutter.

Yes, I had seen Brian drunk, he had seen me drunk, but I never saw Brian falling over or acting splattered like that.

Things have changed now – people are more health-conscious – but back then bands would like to relax after a gig and celebrate their success with a drink.

In that environment, drinking just seemed to be normalised and you build up a tolerance to it, so it doesn't affect you as much. Brian always was on time and organised when working – you would not find him with his head down the loo bowl being sick, so I was, I suppose, able to justify his heavy drinking.

He seemed to be doing okay after his own treatment for skin cancer, but while we were staying in Skegness for four nights where I was performing in *Blood Brothers*, his health started to rapidly deteriorate.

His legs swelled up and he had a painful-looking ulcer on one of them that would not heal.

I begged him to let me cancel my appearance so I could get him home and to a doctor, but he insisted that we carried on as normal and I opened the show.

'I'll be all right, Lin, don't worry about me,' he would say.

But I was worried about him. He was growing more poorly by the hour, never mind the day, and for the first time ever he did not come into the theatre to see the performance as he usually would.

I even told one of my friends, Keith Burns, who played the narrator in the show, 'Keith, I don't think Brian is at all well.'

One morning as I was getting ready to go to the theatre for the matinee performance, Brian told me he was going to take himself off to A&E when I went off to work.

Relieved that he was going to finally see a doctor, I said, 'That's great, Brian. The doctor will be able to sort it.'

He was on my mind all through the performance and as soon as the stage curtain had come down, I rushed back to see him. He tried to make the effort to chat, but it was clear as day to anybody who knew him that he was not himself and I even wondered had he been to see a doctor.

'Did you go to hospital then?' I asked, plonking myself down next to him on the sofa and giving him a cuddle.

'Yeah, Lin, the doctors have given me some painkillers and they've dressed the wound on my leg.'

He showed me and sure enough it had been all cleaned up and bandaged although still grossly swollen.

His face was pained, and I could see he was really struggling, and, for the first time in our professional working partnership, I had to pack up all our stuff from the dressing room and our digs and load up the car.

I didn't mind doing it, but during all our years of working together, it was my job to sing or perform, and Brian would look after everything else.

For instance, if I was booked to play a show in Scarborough for a week, we would book our digs then jump in the Nissan on a Sunday and drive across.

Brian would head off to the venue first without me to check it all out and I would organise our things in our digs or hotel, and then when I would visit the venue for the soundcheck in the afternoon, I would go into my dressing room to find he had

'Brianed' the place, as we jokingly called it. That meant he'd worked his special magic on the place, giving the room a full Brian makeover, transforming it from a bare soulless room to a place filled with flowers and lovely things. There would be platters of fruit and refreshments. Another sweet and thoughtful gesture of his is that he'd bring the good luck cards we got at the beginning of the tour and put them around there, so it was like we had already been there a couple of weeks.

Other performers who happened to come in and see it would say, 'I want a Brian!' I was a lucky woman, I thought, as I tidied everything away and loaded up the car for our journey back to Blackpool; Brian had really spoilt me.

Looking back now on events, I think Brian must have discharged himself from the hospital in Skegness, because he was so poorly; no doctor would send him out in that condition.

And he would have done it for me. Brian would never let me be stuck in a place with no family or friends there to help me, so even though he was seriously ill, he must have walked out of the hospital and used whatever reserves of energy he had left to make sure we got back to Blackpool safely where my family and friends were to rally around us.

My friend Keith from the show also travelled part of the way back with us.

It was a relief to be home, but Brian's leg pain was so bad he was struggling to walk, and I had to help him into the house and onto the couch.

I brought a foot stool over and helped prop his leg up on it so he would be more comfortable. He looked a sorry state and he told me that in the morning, while I was in hospital having my Herceptin treatment, he would go around to the accident and emergency department and have the ulcer on his leg looked at again.

'That's brilliant, Brian,' I told him but inside I felt anxious with worry as I had never seen him this poorly and didn't know what to do.

At that point Keith phoned me and he asked me, 'Lin, did you get home okay? How is Brian feeling?'

I went into another room so we could talk privately and told him, 'I'm worried sick about him, Keith, but I don't know what it is. Brian says he's going to see a doctor in the morning so I will just have to wait until then.'

'I'm glad he's going to see a doctor, Lin,' Keith told me, 'because he was saying some very strange things on the drive home that were out of character, and he wasn't his normal self.'

I thanked him for checking on Brian. Shortly after I hung up the phone, Graham and Sue came around our house to say hello.

I let them in, but Graham could not hide his worry when he clapped eyes on Brian.

'How are you, Brian?' he asked him. 'You don't look great.'

Brian nodded weakly in agreement. 'I don't feel great, Graham, but I'll be okay. I'm going to go to A&E in the morning.'

Quick as a flash, Graham stepped in and told him, 'Er, no, you're not, Brian. You need to go to A&E right now with me. Come on, I'm taking you in.'

Thank goodness he was there and said it. Brian was rapidly deteriorating; he didn't have the energy to put up a protest, so

I went and grabbed my coat and things. Helping Brian get his coat on to go outside, he stopped me.

'Lin, just let Graham take me down now initially and get me sorted because if you're there then I'm just going to worry about you. Stay here, please, with Sue,' he said pleadingly.

I was worried sick and hated the thought of him being there in A&E without me, but I had to respect his wishes. I kissed Brian goodbye and said, 'Okay, give me a call if you need anything.'

Sue waited with me as Graham helped him into the car. As they drove away to the hospital, I tried not to cry, telling myself it was going to be okay, and that he would be home again soon.

Later that evening Graham called me to tell me Brian had been admitted as a patient. I said, 'Oh, okay, thanks Graham for keeping me informed. When can I come down to see him?' And Graham said, 'Lin, the nurse says you should come down to see him immediately.'

I went, 'Oh shit', because as soon as somebody tells you to get to a hospital you know it's serious.

When I arrived at the assessment ward they'd placed him in, it was obvious that, in the few hours since he'd left the house, Brian was growing worse, not better.

While I was trying to hide the fear and worry on my face, Brian was also doing his best to put a brave face on things, telling me he already felt better now he was in hospital and being investigated.

As we were chatting, one of the nurses doing the rounds came in to take his bloods and measure his blood pressure but on seeing the result she legged it out of the room.

As I said to Brian, 'Where the hell did she go running off to like that?', she was suddenly back, bringing about four other nurses and doctors with her.

She told them Brian's blood pressure reading and it was so abnormal he was in danger of having a heart attack.

Suddenly I felt lost and didn't know what to do. I loved him more than anything in the world, he was my soulmate and the thought of anything happening to him was simply inconceivable to me.

You see, Brian was the one who took care of things, he was always there and just knew what to do, and I couldn't imagine my life without him there by my side. He was my world.

Fortunately, they managed to get it under control and once his stats were stabilised the hospital advised me to go home and get some rest and come back in the morning.

As I greeted Brian the following morning his first thoughts were for me and not himself. He asked, 'You will do the show tonight, won't you?' as I was supposed to be getting ready to open *Blood Brothers* at the Palace Theatre in Manchester that night.

'No, Brian, I can't leave you when you're in hospital. I'm going to call them and explain what's happened.'

But Brian was having none of it. Ever the professional when it came to work, he looked at me and said, 'I'm here anyway and they've stabilised me. Manchester is brilliant, Lin, you have to go and play – the press is in tonight. And anyway, visitors aren't allowed here in the evening so you have no excuse but to go and do it!'

I saw his point and I knew it would make him happy if I went.

My sister Maureen kindly drove me across to Manchester in the afternoon to do the soundcheck. I did the show, which was a brilliant success, and then my nephew Danny and his girlfriend came to pick me up to take me home.

It's a tradition on the opening night of the theatre to celebrate the start of a new show with a little tipple, so the three of us popped next door for a quick drink and then they dropped me back home.

I was exhausted from the show and stress, but proud I had carried on as Brian wished, and I was looking forward to going to see him in hospital the next morning and telling him all about how it went.

But that never transpired – at 4am I woke up shivering then started vomiting followed by diarrhoea.

Trying not to panic at what was happening to me, especially as I was ill in the house on my own, I phoned Maureen. Luckily at such an early hour, she picked up the phone.

'Hi Mo, I'm so sick,' I cried. 'Please can you help me?'

She came straight over to mine and got a doctor. Turned out I had cellulitis – a skin infection.

It had set in on my left quadrant where I'd had my surgery and I suppose with all the stress and worry of what was going on it really took hold in the skin. I have been hospitalised twice with it over the years following and it's deeply unpleasant; it can be extremely dangerous if left untreated.

This time, instead of hospital, the doctor said he could treat it at home and put me on high doses of penicillin to kill the bacteria in the skin, but because of the serious infection I was not allowed to go to see Brian in case I passed it on.

It was hell not being able to see him. We made do by chatting to each other every day on the telephone. Sometimes he would sound a little confused and woozy and then other times he would talk like his normal self. I made sure to call the hospital in the morning and they would tell me how he'd fared during the night. Then at lunchtime I would call again and they'd tell me what he'd eaten, before I'd speak to him again in the evening.

Graham and Sue rang me the next day after visiting hours to say a nurse had stopped them on the way out the ward and told them that I needed to talk to a consultant.

I was confused by what they meant and told them the nurses had been telling me he was fine and stable so I presumed the doctors had been on top of his treatment.

On hearing from Sue and Graham, I started going out of my head with worry and needed to know what was going on and to be with him.

I wondered who I could call. I phoned up my breast cancer care nurse, Sarah. As soon as I heard her voice I started to cry.

'Linda, whatever is the matter?' asked Sarah.

'Sarah, they won't let me go and see Brian. He's seriously ill, and they won't let me see him,' I sobbed down the phone.

As she always does, Sarah calmed me down, telling me, 'Linda, leave it with me. I'll phone the ward he's on and call you as soon as I have an answer.'

After quarter of an hour Sarah called back. Her voice had an urgent tone to it.

'Linda, can you come down to my office right away, please, because they're going to let you see him.'

'Thank you!' I sobbed with relief and called Coleen, who was already on her way to mine as it was, and so she picked me up and we drove across the town to Sarah's office.

On arrival she gestured for us to take a seat on her sofa and offered to make us a cup of tea – a cup of tea cures everything, in my book – and I was already feeling happier because I was going to be reunited with my husband.

But as Sarah handed me a cup, I could already see by the look on her face it was not going to be good news.

I took a sip of tea, my stomach muscles tensing in anticipation and fear at the news I knew was about to be served.

'Linda, do you know how sick Brian is?' she asked.

Putting my cup down, I gathered my thoughts and asked her the question I never wanted to hear the answer to. 'Is Brian going to die?'

'Yes.'

Then I remember hearing a high-pitched strange noise coming from somewhere inside the room. I realised the screaming noise was coming from me.

My heart felt like it had been ripped from my chest and the pain was unbearable. Even the simple act of breathing hurt my body. Then next thing Coleen was on her knees in front of me, holding my face in her hands, going, 'Linda, Linda, it's going to be okay, it's going to be okay', as I sat there sobbing and shaking.

When I managed to calm down and get control, I told her: 'Take me to him now, I need to see Brian.'

Sarah swiftly led us along the ward corridor to his bed. As it always did, from the first time that I'd set eyes on him, my heart skipped a beat on seeing him.

It seemed like he was drifting in and out of sleep, but he was aware of my presence as I took his hand and sat beside him.

The consultant came around to his bedside and told me that he was very poorly, and they were doing all that they could for him.

I thanked him, then called Brian's children Lloyd and Sarah to tell them that their father was in hospital. They live in London and I didn't want to alarm or worry them until it was necessary. I explained he was seriously ill and that they should come to see him, and then I rang his best mate John Parker, who lives in Brighton, to deliver the horrible news.

He was driving on the M25 southbound when I called him, and he later told me that when he hung up, he just took the next exit and drove straight back up north to Blackpool.

We were not sure Brian would recognise him, given how ill he was, but when John walked in, Brian's face lit up with joy on seeing him.

'All right, Parkerboy!' Brian managed to say.

For a minute it was like time had stood still between them and they were back to being young men again.

John was thrilled Brian had recognised him because we all knew by then what direction this was heading.

If you are wondering why Brian called John Parkerboy, it's because my husband and his best friend had these nicknames for each other. Brian called John Parkerboy and his name for Brian was Joyceyboy because my mother-in-law was called Joyce and she was the boss in their family. Joyce was a stickler for everything being in the right place and Brian had inherited his mother's brilliant organisational skills, which was what made us such a good working team.

Then his children arrived. It felt very emotional seeing them all together and they gave him a kiss and it was lovely for him to know we were all there with him and he was not alone.

The doctors made sure he was comfortable, and my brothers and sisters went home. John stayed with my brother Brian, and Lloyd and Sarah stayed with me at my house.

I told the youngsters, 'Now don't be sat up late chatting. Please go to bed because we might get a call in the night to go back down and you need to be ready.'

They promised me they would turn in and I went off up to get some sleep myself.

Around 2.30am the hospital rang to tell me they couldn't stabilise Brian and I was to get to the hospital immediately.

I came out my room to give to knock on the doors of his children's bedrooms to tell them to get up, we were needed at the hospital, when I heard lots of chattering and noise coming from downstairs.

They'd ignored what I'd told them and had stayed up talking through the night!

I was already upset as it was and phoned Coleen and told her.

I was angry more than anything at that point, thinking, why could you not just have done what I asked you and gone to bed? Coleen understood my hurt and said she was on her way.

She could see from the cross look on my face and by the atmosphere in the house that I was upset that they had stayed up talking instead of getting some sleep so they would be ready to deal with what was to come at the hospital.

Realising my hurt, they sheepishly asked if they should get a cab and follow us down.

'I don't care what you do,' said Coleen. 'Just get yourselves ready quickly and come to the hospital.'

On the drive over there I was a wreck, wondering what state Brian was going to be in. Coleen did her best to try and soothe my nerves, but when I reached his bedside, I was greeted by a frightening scene.

There were about four or five nurses and doctors trying to get a cannula into his arm. He was vomiting blood and there was so much of it everywhere it looked like he was bleeding out of his skin.

A very dour consultant rushed out to talk to me, and explained they were going to perform a procedure to try to stop the bleeding by putting some stitches in his oesophagus.

'Oh God, he hated that camera going down his throat the last time and said he would never have anything down there again. Is there anything else you can try?' I implored the consultant.

Brian's adult children arrived a few minutes later and I thought to myself this decision is not only up to me; they're his flesh and blood and they too should have a say in the medical treatment and welfare of their father.

I asked them what they thought was the best thing to do with regards the oesophagus operation.

They looked at each other and concluded that as I was Brian's wife and next of kin it was for me to ultimately decide on behalf of their father. However, before I even had the chance to give my response, the consultant – who I nicknamed Medicine Man due to him having some sort of personality bypass – interrupted and said: 'Well, actually it's up to me and we have to do this operation.'

Seeing my crumpled face as a result of the consultant's brusqueness, one of the nurses pulled me to one side and said 'If we don't do this Brian will bleed to death and that's a terrible way to die.'

At this I nodded in agreement and turned back to Brian's bedside to tell him I loved him.

'I love you, Lin,' he managed to mouth to me.

As the nurses prepared to move Brian to the operating theatre, I implored them to call me as soon as there was any news.

So, there we were left together, Brian's children, John, Coleen and me, wandering like lost souls up and down the corridor as there was nowhere for us to sit.

Coleen sensibly suggested our group decamp to the hospital canteen where all the rest of the family could meet us and we could at least get coffees or something to eat if people felt hungry.

We trooped en masse along to the soulless canteen and went through the motions of ordering food and coffee, but I felt so sick I could not swallow a thing or even think about eating or drinking. The pressure and stress started to build up inside me like a pot boiling on the stove, and I began to shake.

Within seconds I was having what can only be described as a full-blown panic attack. My chest felt like an iron band was squeezing it tight and I struggled to get my breath. By this point the rest of my family had arrived and my sister-in-law Annie grabbed a paper bag for me to steady my breathing. Just as my panic subsided, my phone rang.

'Mr Hudson is out of surgery,' said the voice. 'They are bringing him back to the ward once he is stable. Please allow for around twenty minutes before you come to visit him.'

I put the phone down and burst into tears.

'What's happened?' asked the group in unison. 'Is he okay?'

Wiping the tears from my face, I smiled at them and said, 'He's made it through the operation. They're stabilising him and they say we will be allowed to go back to see him in about twenty minutes when they've brought him back up from recovery.'

Everybody breathed a sigh of relief and came across to hug me.

'He's still fighting hard,' I told myself.

But just as I allowed myself a moment of optimism and hope that all was not lost the phone went again.

'I'm so sorry, Mrs Hudson, but you need to come back to the ward right away,' spoke a female voice.

'Sorry, but I don't understand, you just called me a few minutes ago, telling me to wait twenty minutes before coming back. What's going on?' I asked.

'Mrs Hudson, we're sorry … we can't stabilise him—'

Not even giving the nurse the chance to say any more, I hung the phone up and yelled to the others to run to the ward.

We sprinted as hard as we all could, Lloyd, Sarah, John and I followed by the rest of the family.

Just as we got to the curtains surrounding Brian's bed, a nurse came out and announced Brian had died.

I knew by the look on her face what she was going to say.

'I'm very sorry but your husband died a few minutes ago,' she announced.

The next moment was something of a blur. All I remember is that my legs gave way with the shock and I just collapsed into Coleen's arms, sobbing.

The pain in my chest was horrific and my heart kept breaking in two as memories of him and me began flashing through my mind. It just was not possible to imagine my world without Brian in it.

'I need to see him!' I cried.

He looked so peaceful and serene, like he was just asleep and dreaming, and all the stress and trauma of the last few weeks had left his face.

'Oh, Brian, my love,' I exclaimed, and climbed up on the bed beside him, putting my arms around him.

Brian was my first love and the love of my life. My sisters and friends sometimes would ask me, 'How can you be together all the time, Lin?' Or they would joke, 'I would kill whoever it was if they didn't go out to work.'

But for me the days were never long enough as I could not bear being apart from Brian and wanted to spend every hour I had with him. He was my soulmate.

Lying beside his body, I wasn't sure if minutes or hours passed by as time had simply lost all meaning to me.

Eventually, my thoughts were broken by one of the nurses who came across and gently asked if they would be allowed to tidy things up.

Holding on to Brian, I told them I wasn't ready to let go, but my family came over and said: 'Come on, Linda, let us all go outside for a little while so the nurse here can get Brian ready for you and get some air.'

I complied but as soon as they said it was okay to go back in, I just climbed immediately back onto the bed and cuddled Brian again.

Then something very strange happened. When we first arrived at the hospital they asked me what religion Brian was and I said Church of England and they asked if he would like to see a priest? I said no thank you, and that was that.

When he died my Catholic upbringing came to the fore and I shouted "get a priest" he needs the Last Rites.

Well, the chap that turned up at Brian's bedside looked more like a comedian who had dressed up for the day as a funny priest than a real man of the cloth.

He was very skinny, wearing little round spectacles on the end of his nose and was what I would describe as eccentric in appearance.

He started off doing the anointing of the oil and just as I was beginning to give him the benefit of the doubt that he was kosher, he turned to me and asked, 'Are you the Nolan that's in *The Bill*?'

I replied, 'No, I'm the Nolan who's just lost her husband!'

You could not write this stuff, it was that bizarre. I was incredulous that somebody could think and ask such a silly insensitive thing to a person whose partner has just died.

I could see his kids trying to hold in the laughter at this caricature of a priest; Brian would have absolutely loved it and found it hysterical too. It felt like something out of *Spinal Tap*.

My brother came in, took one look at me, and went, 'Lin, you're exhausted. Let's go back to my house.'

Every part of me ached, but I didn't want to leave Brian. The thought of leaving him at the hospital for the last time and going home without him broke me.

'Please, let me stay a little longer. I'm not ready to let go of him.'

Eventually, I said my goodbyes and left, sobbing, as I walked to my brother's car.

I was 22 when I married him, and he was my husband for 26 years. He was 13 years older than me and I was his third wife, so I think he got third time lucky.

· · ·

Back in the house without Brian, my world just fell apart. He'd been the one out of the two of us who had done the organising of events and things, but now it was my turn to be in charge, and

I had to keep it together to arrange his funeral and give him a proper five-star send-off.

It may sound a little morbid, but, as funerals go, friends to this day tell me Brian Hudson's was the best funeral they have ever been to.

Brian himself would have loved it.

The funeral had a concert theme, so all invited guests who came to the church received a lanyard pass to hang around their necks that said 'Brian Hudson's Farewell Tour', just like what you would get when you go to a concert or gig as a special invited guest.

And I gave all the family special 'VIP Access All Areas' passes, like they would have been given to wander around backstage after a concert or to get into an afterparty.

Choosing my husband's coffin was not a pleasant task as the process brought it home again to me that my beloved had left.

The funeral directors were brilliant and worked with me on finding the right coffin design, as I said I wanted his coffin to look like a flight case with DO NOT OPEN and FRAGILE written on it, so it looked like a touring case for a musician's instruments.

When it came to picking what music to be played at the funeral service, you may think two musicians would have difficulty narrowing down their music choices as there are so many great songs with special meaning that we know and love.

Well, it was easy choosing the music for Brian's arrival and departure.

He loved the song 'There You'll Be' by Faith Hill from the film *Pearl Harbor* as it had great meaning to us.

A radio station had played it when we were driving one day and I told Brian that I wanted the song played at my funeral, but Brian went, 'No, no, I want that at my funeral, Lin.'

'Well, you know what, whoever dies first gets it,' I joked back, and we ended up laughing as we were fit and healthy with no thoughts of dying young in our minds.

It quickly became our song, but Brian won and in line with his wishes he got to have his own way at the end.

I felt sick the morning of the funeral, and arriving at the church and seeing all the people that had come to say goodbye to Brian was overwhelming but also uplifting.

Their support and love for Brian gave me a strength to keep going and I could almost feel Brian there with me in spirit, willing me to make it through the day.

We walked in to Faith Hill's song just as Brian would have wished.

The overture was the priest talking as the coffin was brought in and then we had a section called 'fan letters' read out by family and friends in place of tributes.

John or 'Parkerboy', as Brian called him, paid a moving tribute.

My Nephew Jake read a letter I had written to Brian, after all I was his biggest fan!

My brother Brian did the eulogy and there was a recital of the poem 'Stop all the Clocks' by W H Auden.

Brian had been a drummer in a band called Harmony Grass, who'd produced a song years back called 'Move in a Little Closer, Baby'. It had ended up becoming a huge hit, and I chose it as the funeral song to lead his coffin back out of the church.

I asked the six pallbearers who were doing the lifting and carrying of his coffin if they would wear Brian's band T-shirts with his name written on them under their jackets.

As the service drew to a close, they removed their jackets to show off the T-shirts, and when the chorus part of Brian's song played, they lifted him up and carried out his coffin to his song ringing out through the church.

It was beautiful and I could hardly see through my tears, but the love in that room got me through.

Brian had stated he was to be cremated and at the crematorium my sister Denise gave another eulogy. We finished with people walking out to the well-known sounds of 'Always Look on the Bright Side of Life' from the famous Monty Python film *Life of Brian*.

It was a song Brian adored, and everybody went out whistling the tune – even the priest!

So, it was pretty amazing, incredible and uplifting as funerals go, but at the same time horrendous because a funeral is the final farewell, and I was saying goodbye forever to my beloved husband. Getting in the funeral car to go to the wake, I looked back and wondered, whatever will I do now?

ANNE

I was married to my former husband, Brian Wilson, for 27 years. My wedding day to Brian in 1979 was one of the happiest days of my life and we had a loving and happy marriage while it lasted.

Brian is from Newcastle upon Tyne and they have a beautiful accent known as Geordie.

He would call me pet – a popular term of endearment used in the north east of England. I loved it when he called me that and hearing him talk with this gorgeous accent.

He was a professional footballer and only 19 when we met, but due to injury he had to give up his career and retrain as a financial advisor while I was fighting my cancer the first time round.

As I said at the start of this diary, Brian was my rock during my cancer diagnosis and recovery. He was the glue that held our family together. I never heard him once complain or moan or show any signs of feeling sorry for himself, and I don't know what I would have done without him back then as he was a marvellous father to our two daughters growing up.

We went everywhere together. We did everything together, and – because I loved football and with Brian being a footballer – we went to all the football matches together.

He was always doing everything he could to try and look after me – driving me to all my appointments. He came with me to every single chemotherapy session – never missed one – and we would sit together, and he would hold my hand the whole time.

As well as taking me in and out of hospital, he was also looking after the kids, getting them dressed, and taking them to school. The same thing happened when he came to all my radiotherapy appointments. He was there for me and present in my life and in our children's lives – a fantastic husband and parent.

We were a close family, and he was what I would call a proper family man who wanted to do well by his family.

We would go to friends' parties and bring our children, and I would say at a certain point, 'It's late, Brian, I'll take the kids home and you stay here and have another drink.'

But he never ever did; he always came home with me.

When I woke from my lumpectomy operation, his kind face was the first face I saw, and I never doubted his love for me, not for a second.

We went through all of that together and when I was hospitalised for a week during my chemotherapy due to an infection, he just stepped in, got on with it and did the things that needed to be done at home.

I was full of admiration for him. He was amazing.

Linda used to say she could not imagine her life without her own husband Brian in it; well, I felt the same about my Brian and didn't know what I would do without him.

With all this in mind, I had no reason at that time to think he was struggling in any way. He passed all his exams in finance and started up his own financial services business in order to provide for the family as I couldn't work during the cancer treatment. However, the business started to have problems before having to be shut down and he went through a huge personal struggle because of the pressure that he was under, trying to hold the family together and earn a living so we could eat. While I find it difficult going over old things like this, I have to be honest.

He never spoke to me about how he was feeling, and probably most likely he didn't talk to anybody else about it either; in those days men didn't discuss their feelings, and he was having to look after me, having to look after the kids at the same time, and I just don't think he ever asked any of our extended family for help but instead tried to carry on doing it all on his own.

Brian was not a vociferous man, so I didn't notice the beginning of him struggling as he was still the same man – thoughtful and quiet. It started around a couple of years after my treatment finished and I was having quarterly mammograms.

Brian was very funny; he used to make us all laugh with the things he did and said, and he loved cooking and used to cook for us as well.

And then suddenly all that closeness and laughter stopped, and he really went quiet, hardly talking at all.

I thought, something is happening here, but I can't quite put my finger on what it is. He's maybe quiet because he's worried about me, I kept telling myself – me being selfish, assuming he was thinking about me.

And I would push the niggling worries out of my head, remembering what a fantastic husband he'd been throughout my cancer, and kept telling myself that everything's going to be okay.

He didn't talk to me about what was going on because he was trying to protect me. He never said to me, Anne, I'm struggling, and he kept secret from me the horrendous debt that was building up from his business going under.

He was doing all he could to keep that from me while I'm going along in my life, thinking everything's all hunky-dory, but the secret was taking its toll on him and he was under more and more pressure trying to stay afloat without me finding out the truth.

As a couple we didn't argue. I think we may have had one argument in the 27 years that we were together and sometimes I wonder if we might have stayed together if we'd argued a bit more.

There were things clearly bothering Brian and he never let it out because he probably thought we would argue about it and he didn't want us to argue.

27 years is a long time in show business especially as we were apart quite a lot of it, but from my point of view because I thought he was happy I didn't think we needed to argue anymore because things always seemed fine to me.

Now I know that keeping things bottled up and not getting it off your chest is damaging. If he had said the things that were upsetting him and we thrashed it out then it might have saved our marriage.

As it was it didn't get said and had we talked about it and gone to counselling who knows.

But back then things continued to unravel in our marriage, with Brian growing more distant from us all. The atmosphere at home felt strained as he continued to withdraw from myself and the children, and I couldn't get through to him.

Then one afternoon he announced he was off to see his sister for the weekend back in his home city of Newcastle. He casually dropped into the conversation that he was also giving a lift to friends of ours – a married couple – because they were also going to visit some friends in the region.

Normally I would go with him, but I figured it would do him good to spend time with his sister and have a break for a few days to clear his head.

It would do me some good as well as the atmosphere suddenly lifted at home without Brian's dark distant mood hanging over the place.

He called when he arrived in Newcastle to say how the drive went and when I asked after his friend and his wife he suddenly announced that the husband hadn't gone on the journey, just his wife had accompanied him in the car.

I was upset and angry. I thought Brian was giving a lift to some married friends, not another woman on her own.

I didn't want my husband going away for the weekend with another woman, whether they are good friends or not.

I don't care whether that is old fashioned or not, that is how I felt.

Had I known he was driving a female friend unaccompanied to Newcastle for the weekend I would have said no way, I am not happy about that at all and would have told him in no uncertain terms well don't bother coming back if you go!

After a day or so I tried to phone him, and I couldn't reach him. His phone was switched off.

I started to panic as it wasn't like Brian to not check in and keep in contact with the girls and so I phoned his sister, who told me he'd taken this female friend to see Holy Island, the beautiful tourist landmark in the North Sea.

Holy Island is where Brian and I spent our honeymoon. There was only us and a couple of other people on this tiny island and it was bliss.

You can imagine the special memories it holds for me and at that time I would not have dreamt of going there with another man other than Brian.

Well, a few more days passed as the island has no phone signal. When he finally called me, I calmly asked him if he'd been to Holy Island with this married woman.

He told me, 'Yes, Anne. Her husband couldn't make it so I thought we would go there for a couple of days.'

I thought about the mood swings and how I had felt sorry for him because he seemed so low and was worrying about his wellbeing, then here he is waltzing around on our honeymoon island with another woman in tow. The audacity of it. I shouted, 'Well, don't bother coming home then!', and slammed the phone down.

Well, Brian did come home straight away to try and make amends and he was trying to be nice and talk about it, but I was hurt and it just escalated from there.

I accused him of having an affair with this woman and asked how he could be so insensitive, taking another woman to our special place.

Brian protested and said she was just a friend and reminded me she was his friend's wife and swore nothing had happened, but I was too hurt to listen and told him to get out and he was to leave our house.

He was devastated but agreed to my wishes. He packed up his things and moved into this poky flat around the corner from our house so he could regularly see our daughters.

This was the point Brian's struggles were really starting to take a hold of him but I didn't know at the time what was really going on with him. Looking back now I don't think anything untoward went on with that other woman. I called her up and she was adamant nothing had happened, insisting to me they had not kissed, and they had gone there as friends as she had been trying to support him, because to her Brian seemed in a bad way and she was concerned about him.

And to be fair to Brian, the three of them had been friends for years. Brian used to manage a local football team when he gave up professionally and their son had played on one of the teams, so they would hang out after the matches and go for drinks and stuff.

Interestingly, her husband was also fine with it all. He believed his wife when she said nothing happened between them, and he believed Brian and they are still friends as far as I know.

I now believe Brian wasn't having an affair with her, but it was the catalyst for him to leave our marriage. In time he became happy in his new place and he met somebody else. And, of course, when I found that out, I wanted him back straight away.

I went over there and said, 'Brian, I want you to come back. Please come home!'

He shook his head, saying no, he wouldn't come back and there were certain things that had happened he couldn't ever get over.

It wasn't until after we were divorced, and I read the divorce papers and his statement, I found out his exact reasons, which shall remain private.

However, I thought well you never said any of that when we were together.

If he had said it, we could have talked about it and even gone to counselling and he might not have left in the long run, but I don't know, maybe it wasn't meant to be.

But back at the time, the split didn't stop me doing what I could to save us. I went round to his place and told him that I still loved him, begging him to come back, suggesting we go to counselling together to try and sort it out.

It was just before our 25th wedding anniversary as well and the things he was telling me didn't make any sense, and with no disrespect I don't think he knew what the hell he was doing or saying at that moment in time.

And then the inevitable happened and he met another woman who helped him through it. She's an auxiliary nurse, and apparently when I was having my chemo at the hospital, she used to chat to him, which helped him get through things, and give him support.

They ended up getting married, and they're still together. I don't have any grievance against Brian because he was an amazing husband and he was there by my side when I most needed him – helping and supporting me during cancer – and he was a brilliant father to our children.

I don't what I would have done without him back then and until our relationship stopped working, we had a fantastic marriage, we really did.

What made things hard was that we had two daughters to think about.

I wish my marriage had lasted. That's one thing that I would really love to have happened, but it didn't and I can't really change it.

I was a bit of a lunatic during our divorce because divorcing is painful, but I hold no bitterness or regrets. I concentrate on all the good parts now.

All you can do is pick up the pieces and start to move on with your life.

CHAPTER 6

THE AFTERMATH

LINDA

After the funeral, my world started to fall apart. All I could think about from the minute I woke to the moment I closed my eyes again was Brian.

When asked, I would tell people I was 'fine', but I was nothing of the kind.

Eating, watching TV, or just the simple task of getting out of bed, washing my hair, and putting on some clothes held no appeal for me and seemed utterly pointless.

I didn't want to go out or eat, so for the next six weeks I stayed in and my sisters as ever were marvellous, and took it in turns to stay at my house and care for me despite my protestations that I didn't need anything or anybody.

'Come on, Linda, try and eat a little something. You need to keep your strength up.'

And I would try to force some food down before heading back to bed. I became a queen of daytime napping and lost track of the hours and days.

Denise came into my bedroom one afternoon while I was dozing.

'Linda, are you awake?'

My eyes flickered open and I could see from her stance she meant business.

'Listen, Lin,' she said, 'there's little creatures knocking on my door saying, can you change Linda's sheets? Whether we have to peel you off the bed or whatever, we need to change those sheets!'

'I don't feel like getting up,' I told her.

'Linda, we're all very worried about you … please let me help you. The others tell me you haven't been out the house since the funeral. You can take a shower, put some clean pyjamas on, and I will have it all cleaned up and fresh linen on by the time you come out. You will sleep much better tonight on clean sheets.'

'I'm tired and being here makes me feel close to Brian; I can still smell his scent on the pillow. It's all I have,' I told her. 'Please don't wash it away.'

I closed my eyes, thinking if I didn't look at her she would get the hint and leave me be, alone with my thoughts.

It didn't work and Denise sat on the end of the bed. I shifted position away from her to hug Brian's pillow, inhaling his familiar warm and comforting smell.

'I'm fine, Denise. You don't have to change them for me; I promise I will do it tomorrow,' I tried telling her, hoping she'd take the hint and leave me to sleep.

But Denise wasn't buying my promise and realising this was not a battle I was going to win and seeing sense in the end I heaved myself off the bed and went into the bathroom.

Looking at myself in the mirror I knew I had stopped caring about myself, stopped caring in general about everything that had once mattered to me. It all seemed so meaningless now Brian wasn't with me to share it.

Every step was an effort like climbing a high wall but never reaching the top.

My heart was broken, and it showed. My face looked pale with dark circles under red swollen eyes due to broken nights crying, while my limbs felt heavy under the weight of grief.

In the shower I stood under the hot water for ages. It felt good letting it pound down on me washing my tears away. When I came out, the bed was changed. It wasn't that I actually wanted to sleep in dirty sheets forever more… of course not. The reason I had kept them on there for so long was that I felt close to Brian in our bed. Smelling his essence on the pillows made it feel he was still there beside me in some capacity and washing them was like washing Brian away with them.

To remind myself of him I started spraying his aftershave on the pillow before going to sleep.

Brian used to wear Fahrenheit aftershave by Christian Dior and to this day I still sometimes spray the scent because I find it comforting.

What I've learned over the years of dealing with grief is that when people lose somebody they love, they react in all kinds of different ways.

Some people clear out the deceased person's wardrobes of the clothes or belongings straight away. I had a friend who did it on the day her husband died. She had to get rid of his clothes immediately because they just brought her down again.

My belief is everybody should be allowed to grieve how they wish to do so. There is no right way or wrong way or right or wrong time. It is what feels right to you.

I didn't clear out Brian's wardrobe for more than two years. I tried on many occasions to go through his things, saying to various friends if they were visiting, 'Come on, let's do the wardrobe today.'

Then I'd go upstairs full of good intentions, open the wardrobe to see Brian's clothes hanging there, only to turn around and say, 'Oh, let's not', and we would go sit back downstairs and it would go back on the 'things I will get around to doing' list for another day.

At that time, the barrier stopping me from clearing out his clothes was the same as not washing the bedding. I thought clearing away his things would feel like losing him all over again.

Then one day after two and a half years, when my friend happened to be visiting me, I got up from the chair and said to her, 'Come on, let's go upstairs and do this.'

We grabbed a load of empty bags and raced upstairs to the bedroom before I had the opportunity to change my mind. This time when I pulled open the wardrobe doors there was no little voice in my head telling me, 'No, Linda, you're not ready.' And so, we began …

It was a big job clearing out Brian's clothes as he had built up quite a collection over the years.

As we folded them up and packed them away it brought back memories of nights out, holidays and wonderful times. Brian loved wearing suits and had an array of them squashed into the wardrobe.

If I were working in a cabaret club Brian would always dress up in a lovely suit and coloured tie in the evening. He looked great in a suit, I thought, very smart and handsome.

At one stage my friend pulled another of Brian's sartorial choices out the wardrobe and started laughing.

'What has you tickled all of a sudden?' I asked her.

'This suit, Linda,' she squealed. 'Look at the size of the shoulder pads in it!'

She paraded it around and I couldn't help it either; peals of laughter erupted from me because it was such an eighties-looking suit with these ridiculous big shoulder pads like an American footballer has – God love him.

It was an emotional task, but my friend was brilliant and really helped me to get through it. We would pack up some clothes, go downstairs and drink some gin, then come back up and tackle it once more until it was finally all done.

At the end, I kept one of his fleeces and a lovely light blue T-shirt. I keep them in a bedding box and I sometimes wear them in bed.

During the months after Brian's death, my doctor diagnosed me with complex grief. I became suicidal and I went in a complete downwards spiral. Subsequently, I was placed under the care of the local mental health crisis team, which meant they could visit twice a day unannounced.

At the time it was a relatively new service, which allowed them to treat people like myself with depression at home first rather than in a hospital. I could phone up 24/7 and they would come out to my house if I needed them. They were amazing.

My diagnosis came about through the therapy sessions I had with Dr Jean Brigg, the psychologist I had started to talk to when I was diagnosed with my cancer. She had saved my life on several occasions by talking to me and making me realise that things – when you look at them in a different light – can be different.

Now, I was desolate because Brian wasn't here, and I could not see a life without him. As much as I could, I would try and go out, but then I'd come home, shut the front door and slide down the wall, thinking of ways to end my life. I was also financially struggling because I hadn't worked, and I wasn't well.

During one of my therapy sessions, things came to the boil. I was angry, sad and didn't know what to do. When I got home my phone was ringing and my GP was on the phone, telling me she was worried about me and wanted to give some support. She said, 'Your psychologist phoned me and wants me to refer you to the mental health crisis team.'

I hung up and was so angry I phoned the psychologist and left a message on her answerphone: 'You snitch!'

Anyway, they sent this female psychiatrist to assess me, and she brought two men with her, who I think were nurses. They hung around in the background while I spoke to the doctor.

During that first visit I told the psychiatrist the truth about how I was really feeling. 'I look out of the window and there is no hope, there is no light at the end of the tunnel. I think everybody would be happier knowing I was with Brian and they would understand,' I explained.

There was no holding back once I started to speak and I let her know how hard it was, admitting I even had written a goodbye letter, starting with the words, 'I know you will understand …' to all my sisters and brothers.

It sounds shocking now that I had done that, but at the time I convinced myself that my family would understand if I chose to take my own life because six months had passed, and I was still crying.

'I bet when my name comes up on the phone, they go, it's Linda, don't answer it,' I cried to her, hot tears of hurt and anger bubbling up from inside me.

Of course, I know that's not the case under any circumstances, and how my family would be extremely hurt and upset if they thought that was what I was thinking about them. However, at the time, when you are in the middle of an episode as I was, things look different; the only way I can explain it to non-sufferers of clinical depression is that the negative thoughts are so overwhelming, they drown out your inner voice of reason.

At the time I had my beloved pet dog, a Bichon Frise dog called Hudson (he passed on 17 August 2015), and in the letter, I also put, 'PS Please, look after Hudson.' When I finished getting everything off my chest, I took another look at the two men with her and suddenly had a thought, maybe they were there to catch me and carry me away into hospital if I tried to protest and escape out the door.

Truth was this doctor didn't need the big men with her that day. I was so low I wouldn't even have put up a finger at them in defence if she said they were taking me with them. Grief had overwhelmed my mind and body to such an extent that I would have said yes to going with them anywhere if it meant an end to all the pain, hopelessness, and feelings of despair I had been carrying.

Leaning forward slightly in the chair, she spoke gently to me, 'Linda, you've got nothing to lose but to let us try and if it doesn't help and you don't feel better then nobody can stop you doing what you want to do, but I think we can help you because I think your grief has gone over into clinical depression.'

'Okay then, whatever,' I told her, slumped in my seat. 'Do what you want.'

The psychiatrist didn't take me into hospital that day, but she did prescribe me a course of anti-depressants. While it didn't make my depression go away overnight, under her brilliant care and the prescribed medication I could finally manage what I was feeling.

The tablets combined with therapy with Dr Brigg meant I would wake up in the mornings and not cry. They were literally a lifeline as I started to find living easier to deal with.

During that treatment protocol I was able to phone them in a panic to say I'm really struggling, and while they couldn't always get back to you straight away, you could leave a message and the secretary was great at getting back to you and making an appointment.

Years down the line I told my brothers and sisters about the goodbye letter I had written them, and my brothers said to me, a) 'None of us would understand so take that with you', and b) 'none of us are having the dog and so we know you won't do it now because of the dog'!

I know, despite everything I've gone through since, that I will never go back to that dark place.

My counselling sessions really were a lifeline that helped me to look at things in new ways.

If Dr Brigg had said to me, 'Linda, I'm going to pass you on to another psychologist', I would have been bereft because she had been my touchstone from when it all started with my cancer the very first time. I would have told her I can't do it again with somebody else because it'll just bring me back to a place that I don't want to be reliving it all again from the beginning.

You build up an amazing trust with somebody and you can start to think they're like a friend. When you're discharged, the funny thing is you end up thinking: they didn't even phone! You can become dependent on people and with all the clinicians I see, I realise the relationship is a patient–professional one. They are doing a job. They know everything about my life, but I know nothing about their lives; they are brilliant at their jobs and instil this trust in you that they are there to help you, which of course they are.

Through the therapy sessions I began to realise that clothes and possessions are inanimate objects. Brian's in my heart and nobody will ever take that away. If I lost everything, even now, I would still have Brian.

However, before I got the treatment to make me better, it was a really difficult time and I suffered terrible paranoia. I booked and paid for five holidays that year and went on none of them because when it got close to the time of travelling, this fear would take hold that paralysed me from doing anything or going anywhere.

I can't even explain what the fear actually was; maybe it was fear of change, fear of something happening when I was away and not being able to control it, fear of doing something or enjoying myself without Brian with me. However, grief is not rational, and its grip was so strong it would render me powerless, and just as the flight time drew near, I would turn around and say, 'I can't go away', losing all the money I'd shelled out for the trip and saying sorry to others for pulling the holiday at the last minute.

Dr Brigg suggested one day the great idea that some of them came with me to one of my therapy sessions with the psychiatrist to see what was involved and hear what we talk about, and maybe in doing so get to understand a little bit more of what I was going through.

I chose Maureen and Coleen to come with me. Initially it felt a little odd having them in the room with me, but within a few minutes I chatted away freely with no self-censorship.

I had even forgotten they were there until the psychiatrist turned to them and said, 'Ladies, do you wish to ask Linda any questions?'

Turning to me, Mo asked, 'Linda, why don't you just say you don't want to go away? Why go through with the pretence of booking the holidays when you don't want to go?'

'It's because I feel I should, and I know I should,' I told her.

Through therapy I now know putting pressure on yourself to do something because you think you should – when in actual fact you're not ready – does not work.

At the end, Dr Brigg asked Maureen for her thoughts on the session and if she had any questions for her?

'It's helped me to realise it's not just a quick fix and "oh, get over yourself!", Maureen announced. She was very sympathetic and, at that time, I felt she understood my predicament and state of mind more than Coleen.

Asked for her thoughts on the counselling session, Coleen was a little more blunt, shall we say, than Mo.

'I could not do your job because I would want to give them a kick up the bum and tell them "get out there, you can do it", she told them.

But the psychiatrist, quick as a flash, replied, 'Yes, you clearly couldn't do my job!'

That did make me laugh.

Another example of the difference between their two approaches towards my management of my grief was when I was offered a role in a play.

The first panto I did away from Brian was in Worthing, where I played the Wicked Queen. In between shows I got a call from my agent saying I had been offered a part in the play *Grumpy Old Women*, which would be staged in Ireland.

It was great money, and it would pay my expenses such as my accommodation and travel costs. Pre-cancer and losing my husband I would have jumped at the opportunity.

But, again, the fear that stopped me going on those holidays set in once more and I could not face travelling to Ireland. Emotionally I could not be away from everybody, it was too hard, but I didn't want people to think I was a failure because I could not do it.

I asked my agent for a few hours to make up my mind and I phoned up the nurse at the lymphoedema clinic who did the bandaging on my arms to help suppress the swelling, and told her about the acting offer I had received, which meant moving to Ireland for an interim.

She said she could arrange for me to have the bandaging done at a hospital over there, but deep down it wasn't the answer I wanted to hear.

I knew in my heart I was not ready for this step and had wanted her to tell me it was not possible, so I had a legitimate excuse to give to the agent as to why I was turning it down.

So, I was honest, and I said to her, 'I don't want to go, though,' and she said: 'Well, tell them you can't go because we've got to see you!'

I thanked her and put the phone down then called up my sister Bernie in tears and told her about the offer, how amazing it all was, but the nurse said I didn't have to go if I didn't want to and I didn't know what to do for the best.

Bernie, who never judged, simply asked me, 'Linda, do you want to go?'

Without hesitation I told her, 'No.'

'Well, don't go then.'

I just needed someone to go, 'it is okay to say no, think about your health'. And that was what Bernie did.

'Oh God, thank you so much', I cried.

I called Coleen and told her about the job offer, but explained, 'I can't go. I can't go, Col.'

'You can, Linda. You can do this,' she urged me, the opposite to Bernie and the hospital nurse. 'You are strong; get out there and do this.'

Coleen is one of those 'gets on and does what she says she's going to do' kind of people, which I admire, and during the call she tried her best to cajole me into action with an energetic 'I know you can do it.'

She was the only one I spoke to who said to go and do the show.

I was rattled by that point, and began to think Coleen could be right, and whether I would be making a big mistake if I didn't go.

The adage that we grew up with – that we carried on working unless on our death bed – was haunting me, and I felt like I was letting myself down.

I needed my mum to put her arms around me and say, 'come home with us' where she would make up a bed on the couch like when I was a kid, but she wasn't there to take the decision out of my hands, so I kept phoning other people searching for others to tell me not to go.

Going over it again in my head I then phoned Maureen, told her everything and she simply said: 'Don't go.'

Maureen echoed what Bernie had said and what I knew was the right thing to do in my heart; I simply was not ready to make that journey without Brian. It was a fabulous offer, but I was just so sad, and I didn't want to be away from home feeling the lonely way that I did.

And with that I called my agent thanking him for the amazing offer but explaining that my illness and hospital treatment prevented me from taking it up. There were no regrets when I said no, only relief.

I found those first few years after losing Brian was a really terrible time – very hard and very difficult. I was capable of making decisions and had made decisions before but during our marriage when I was away working, he made a lot of the decisions at home and that set-up just worked for us that way. Some people will think take control of your destiny and don't be lazy but that was our life. I liked him deciding on things for us when I was busy at work and didn't want to be bothered. Consequently, when he died and I was diagnosed with clinical depression I initially struggled with making decisions such as whether to take a job or not. But I have learned over time and had to grow up if you like. Now I know what I want and can decide for myself.

I don't know if Maureen understood what I was going through more than Coleen, but I think people react to stuff in different ways. In the psychiatrist's office that day, they both said how they felt, and it helped me to realise that they were terribly worried about me and were doing their best to help me in their own different ways.

There were times when I did feel a very lonely, and Annie, my sister-in-law, was amazing and became my buddy because the other girls were all busy working. I could call her and say, 'Will you come round?' and she would be there. My nieces were brilliant also.

I remember the first time I went shopping to do a grocery shop after losing Brian, at my local Tesco, which was a ten-minute walk away. All the way back I sobbed. There was a football match on, which made it worse, as I kept thinking me and Brian would be at the football. It set me off worrying that I took him for granted all the time, as I realised that if there was no milk in, he was the one to go out and get it. He did all the shopping. I never had to think about it because he sorted it. But this led me to thinking: did he know that I loved him?

I said it to the girls, and they all laughed out loud at me.

'What do you mean?' they said. 'You used to go shopping or come to Sainsbury's with one of us and phone him three times or he would phone you three times. You were only getting the bloody shopping! You were both like characters from a Mills and Boon novel.'

Brian was a romantic. For two years I got a dozen red roses every ten days.

The florist would put them in a vase for me, until one day I said to him, 'Bri, they are so beautiful, but we are going away, and we won't get the pleasure of looking at them.'

We both decided the flowers were a waste of money when sometimes we would be going away to work, so we cancelled the order and Brian would turn up with flowers not only on birthdays and anniversaries but just because he loved me.

When he died, I started keeping a single long-stemmed red rose in a vase by the telly for him. After telling the counsellor this, she said to me, 'You know if you come back and the rose has died or you get rid of it, don't feel guilty.'

Another time I couldn't find a ring he bought me, and I was desperate about how I let him down. It put me in such a state of anxiety, and I cried. Eventually to my relief I did find it, but now I look back and can see it doesn't matter because he's always with me.

It was a terrible time for me, it really was as it had a terrible impact on my general health. I tried to go back to work to *Blood Brothers*, but when in Wolverhampton I got cellulitis in my left arm.

When in hospital I asked, 'Do you think this is my body saying, you need to rest?' Maureen and Bernie were doing a play in Lichfield, Staffordshire, called *Mum's The Word*, at the time, but Maureen got her understudy to step in for her and she used my hotel room and she kept watch over me with Bernie, who would also pop over when possible in the day.

At one point the nurse went to give me an injection but she went and nearly injected Maureen, who was asleep on my bed! My brothers were also amazing during that horrible period. They came down to collect me and said, 'where is your bag because we are taking you home.'

A long time after the Wolverhampton incident I went to Bradford to see Mo appear in *Blood Brothers* – she was there all week. After a few days I noticed my arm was red and it started to feel sore.

I showed Mo when she got home from the theatre and she said, 'Let's go to the hospital before it takes hold.'

Cellulitis is so painful that you can't touch your fingers - like a scald. I get flu like symptoms with a raging temperature.

The hospital sent me home that night with a high dose of antibiotics and they drew a circle around the red patch on my arm with the warning if the red patch goes outside the circle come back immediately.

The next morning the red patch had gone way outside the circle and I felt rubbish, so I went back to the hospital where they admitted me and I was put on intravenous antibiotics for a week!

Poor Mo, Bradford was the last week of the tour and she was looking forward to going home, but instead of doing that she stayed so she could visit me in hospital, bless her. I am so lucky to have my brilliant family who have always helped to look after me.

In my profession I'm not used to people saying that, and it made me realise that yes, you have to be kind to yourself sometimes.

The next thing I undertook was my breast reconstruction operation. It came at the time we had fallen out with the girls just after our tour, and I was nervous. Maureen came down to Wythenshawe Hospital to help me get settled in and I brought a picture of Brian and token urn containing some of his ashes.

The nurse thought he was still alive because I had been asking for him as I was coming round from the anesthetic.

She said to Mo, 'who is Brian?' and Mo said 'her dead husband.' The nurse was mortified.

They could only put a little Saline to enlarge my new breast because my skin had lost its elasticity, so to make them even they did another operation to reduce my other breast.

I had a nipple made from my own skin for my new breast but the tissue died and it fell off. The second attempt was successful, thank God!

I managed to get back home just before Christmas and everybody who came to see me, I scared the life out of them by flashing them my new 36C breast!

The scars were neat, and the surgeon who is like a magician in my eyes said I had good elasticity in the skin. When I first checked the bandaged breast area just seeing the shape like my old breast was an incredible emotional feeling and it is like getting part of your old self back.

I was euphoric after everything had settled down and it felt amazing putting on a swimsuit and feeling like me again.

I told the surgeon 'thank you, for giving me back me again.'

· · ·

There is a tendency when a loved one has died to put them up on pedestal and talk about them like they are a saint and I probably did do the same with Brian initially.

He was an amazing husband and Brian and I had a fabulous time, but we were a normal couple who argued like all couples do.

I never mentioned his drinking and that he had died from too much drink because I wanted people to love him like I loved him.

My dad, when he was ill, was a terrible patient to my mum sometimes. She didn't drive and he made her go back to the shops to get certain things he liked and then when he died, my two brothers and I were there, and my mum said to the consultant, 'Oh, he was such a wonderful patient though.'

Our heads went, one after the other, looking at our mum incredulously, going, are we on the same planet here?

It was just so funny, but they had their moments and by later life, they realised how much they loved each other.

When I say Brian spoilt me, he really had, almost to a fault.

I didn't know anything when it came to the house; documents, banking, life admin ... Brian had taken care of it all.

Coleen's former husband Ray, and a great friend of ours Mark Styles came to the house the day after Brian had died and cancelled his phone and credit cards.

They asked me, 'Where are your insurance papers and documents for the car, like your V5 certificate?' And I had to tell them I didn't even know what they were talking about. The only word I recognised with V and 5 in it was a shampoo brand!

Once I left the girls in 1983 Brian left with me he became my manager. We did the gigs together, he would drive and do my sound and it was great. When *Blood Brothers* came along it was difficult for him. As my manager he negotiated the contract and the first one was for 6 months so, in effect his work was done.

Brian felt redundant. I pointed out that I couldn't do the tour without him. I don't drive for start, he took the burden of booking accommodation off me.

He solved any problems that occurred and, as I said earlier he 'Brianed' every dressing room for me!

Remembering that time makes an old conversation I had with Shirley Reid, the wife of comedian Mike Reid, years earlier when Brian was still alive float into my head. Seeing how Brian was looking after everything, she advised me to find out where everything was kept in the house because, without being morbid, Brian wouldn't be around forever, and she could see I was spoilt to a fault. She told me: "You need to sort out where everything is because he is not going to be around forever, Linda." How I wish I'd heeded her advice.

Having learned about these things the hard way, I've passed that information on over the years to other female friends, including my sister Denise who has been with her fiancé of 40 years, Tom for 47 years, telling her: 'Denise, do yourself a favour, would you? Just find out where things are kept? Have a designated place or drawer for all the car documents, insurance papers, deeds to the house and so on, so if anything happens you know where everything is kept and it's in order.'

The paperwork was initially overwhelming, and I would go into my dining room and find letters and documents piled up on the table. The mental health team came in to help me one day make all the phone calls to utility companies and so forth and now I do everything like that myself.

Even now Maureen says 'Oh my God, Linda', because I am so organised. I am in complete control now in what is going on and I have just sorted my credit cards with the help of a Macmillan support worker, Julie Summers, who has been amazing.

When I started to feel lighter in mood, I used to joke to the girls that 'I've done a man job', if I changed a lightbulb or bled a radiator. I'm proud that I've adapted and learned to live and cope on my own. It's not been easy, but I've done it and I love my little house.

I ordered things for my house from Italy on my iPad and when I showed the girls they were so impressed I could do it. I have become quite independent in that respect.

I find the weekends the worst as a single woman. When Brian was alive, we loved our Sundays, going for a walk with the dog or cooking Sunday lunch.

I know if I were to phone my family and say I was on my own they would invite me around, but I don't like to bother them when they are with their families. They need their own family time. I'm just thankful to have them.

And what of Brian's son and daughter. Lloyd is 44, and Sarah turned 50 last year. When they were children, I spent time with them on weekends and they would stay with us in the holidays. When their dad passed, they could have, as stepchildren, loosened off a little bit as their dad wasn't here so they don't have to come and see me, but I'm pleased to say they've been absolutely amazing. They're like my own kids and they've given me grandchildren! I have a granddaughter who is 21 and I have a granddaughter who was seven in January. I've been lucky that Lloyd and Sarah have been so brilliant and are fabulous.

I wanted children. It is my only regret in life that I didn't have children. I always say, I know the kids love me, but when their mum or dad walks in, they get a smile I will never get because I am not their mum and dad, but that's beautiful and under-standable and how it should be because they are their parents. However, it was nobody's fault except my own because I kind of let my career get in the way. We would think about trying and then I'd go, well, we'll have to wait till after we've done this year at Maggie May's or this pantomime.

I try not to dwell on not having my own children with Brian and I've never looked at women with babies, thinking, 'Oh, that could have been me.'

It's more, 'Oh God, what a shame we never did', and the girls always say, 'Out of all of us, Lin, we'd have thought you would have ten kids running around.'

I did investigate fostering babies once upon a time. It was my counsellor that planted the seed into my head after she said to me, 'Linda, the only time I see a light in your eye during our therapy sessions is when you're talking about your great-nieces and -nephews. Just a glimpse of a sparkle of light comes into your eyes when you are talking about the kids. I wondered have you thought about trying fostering?'

After that conversation I went home and started the applica-tion process for fostering, but then Bernie was diagnosed with her cancer and I wanted to see her and spend quality time with her.

Anyway, by the time I came back to the fostering application process the paperwork had mounted up.

It was off-putting how much of it there was – unbelievable amounts. All you want to do is look after a child and make them feel safe and loved, and then this whole bank of paperwork comes in and you think, 'Oh my God, I can't deal with that.'

But I have been blessed with my stepchildren from Brian and their children as well as my nieces, nephews, great-nieces and great-nephews, who bring joy into my life.

What I hope this chapter has shown is the healing counselling gives. If you are in despair or struggling, I say to everybody just try it.

The thing about counselling is, if you don't like it, you don't have to go back but you just have to give it a chance.

It saved my life so many times.

CHAPTER 7

BLUE-EYED GIRL

We had to give our beloved Bernie her own chapter because she is a mammoth part of us and our cancer story.

As we worked together for so long, every single song is a reminder or a memory of Bernie.

During the *The Nolans Go Cruising*, we talked about Bernie a lot. Maureen found it very cathartic to talk things out and Coleen also said she felt like Bernie was with us throughout filming for the cruise show, because to everything we did as a family on that magical trip, we would all go, 'Oh, Bernie would have loved this', or 'Can you imagine if Bernie was here now?'

Bernie would have caused a mutiny on that boat because she was hysterically funny, and everybody who knew her loved her. In this chapter we both relive our memories of our beloved sister, what she meant to each of us, and how we coped with losing her.

Bernie was only 52 when she died and a warrior to the very end. Thousands of fans lined the streets at her funeral in Blackpool, testament to how much she was loved and revered.

Like both of us, her cancer started in her breast, but it was aggressive and quickly spread to her brain, lungs, liver and bones.

2020 would have been her 60th birthday and she would have held the party to end all parties to celebrate joining the 60's club, while drinking her favourite tipple, a Moscow mule – which is vodka, ginger ale and we add a squeeze of fresh lime.

To celebrate the occasion, we had planned a 300-person ball, which we would use to raise money for Cancer Research, but as we were hit by the Covid pandemic no large gatherings were allowed.

Instead, we marked her special day with a socially distanced private dinner, in line with the government guidelines, and gave our own personal tributes. There was a big cake for her and of course we had a picture of her there.

We all said we couldn't imagine her being 60, and we talked about what we think she would be like now.

Before Bernie became sick with cancer, we had a general consensus among us siblings that Bernie was like our Aunty Lily, who'd lived until she was 99 and was five foot nothing.

99! Aunty Lily was just like our Bernie: the life and soul of the party. We used to tease her, saying, 'You're just like our Aunty Lily; you'll be there at ninety with a cigarette (this was before she stopped smoking) knocking back a glass of vodka and you will be the last one up!'

Bernie would laugh; she was a pocket rocket full of insatiable energy and verve.

If you were ever anywhere with Bernie, she would be the last one standing. Even when you would stay at her house and it was 3am and your eyes were closing in front of her, you were that tired, Bernie would say, 'No, you're doing no such thing!', if you'd told her you were going to bed. She would forbid you and you'd end up asleep on the sofa while she nattered away. We used to think with that attitude she would be around forever.

To make it extra special for her 60th in lockdown, we asked fans over social media to celebrate her big day by sending their pictures of their toasts to her.

The large outpouring of love on Twitter/Facebook and Instagram was beautiful and lifted our spirits.

Bernie was a remarkable woman. She was the first of us to start a television acting career with roles on *Brookside* and *The Bill*, and right up until she took her last breath, her personality shone so brightly.

She will never be forgotten because she was too vibrant and big a character for anyone to forget her.

She made such a mark on all of us and the world, and we will never get over losing her; a simply unforgettable sister, mother, aunt, and woman in her own right, who was gone too soon.

We think about and miss her every day and will love her forever.

Anne and Linda x

LINDA

Bernie had spotted in a mirror that her breast did not look right back in the spring of 2010. She had dimpling of the skin and went to have it looked over.

I was in the car with Maureen the day I got the devastating news it was cancer.

She had come to collect me from town where I had been shopping.

Bags in the boot and nestled in the passenger seat with my seatbelt on, we drove off towards my house.

I noticed Maureen seemed rather tense and not her normal cheery disposition and asked her if something was up?

She suddenly pulled over and stopped the car.

'Mo, what is it, why have we stopped?'

Steeling herself for what she was about to say, Maureen took a deep breath.

'Okay, Linda, I need to tell you something and I don't want you to get upset,' she said, but her eyes were beginning to swim with tears before she'd even finished her sentence.

'Mo, are you okay? What has happened?' I heard my voice rise in panic.

'It's Bernie, Lin ... she has been diagnosed with breast cancer,' sobbed Maureen.

Boom! It was like a detonator went off inside me. Physical pain ripped at my insides, just as it had with Brian's diagnosis.

I felt winded from the shock, and could only utter 'Oh, my God' in response.

Bernie, no, it couldn't be true, I thought; it couldn't be. My mind was scrambling to put it together, trying to understand how this came to be. Yes, I'd had cancer, and so had Anne, but Bernie was younger than me. She had a daughter, a wonderful life; she was so beautiful and full of energy. Not our Bernie ... not my lovely funny baby sister.

'When? How?' was all I managed to say, praying Maureen was going to tell me the doctors had caught it quickly and it was curable.

'We all found out a few days ago, but we didn't know how to tell you or what to say. I'm sorry.'

I never spoke, and Maureen continued, 'You've been through such an ordeal, Linda, with your own cancer then losing Brian and well ... Bernie, and us lot, we didn't want to upset or worry you after all you have recently suffered.'

That was Bernie, always thinking of others before herself.

I started to think of Bernie and me as kids. There was only a year and nine months difference in age between us and we had been thick as thieves.

We'd go off to play; we loved making up dances when we were little. Coleen would often join in with us and I found myself smiling at the sweet memories. Happy days back then as children with not a care in the world.

My family knew how close we were as sisters and I understood they were doing their best to shield me from further heartache and pain.

Mo started up the engine to drive me home and I did not say much else the rest of the way for I was in a state of shock and could not think properly.

When she pulled up outside my house, Mo asked if I wanted her to come inside with me and stay for a bit.

'Don't worry, Mo, I'll be fine,' I told her, adding, after seeing her concerned face, 'I'll give you a ring.'

Waving her off at the door I went inside but no sooner than I'd shut it behind me, I thought, 'Oh my God, I can't bear it', and slid down the wall onto the floor.

Lying there in a crumpled heap, sobbing my heart out, I felt angry that this was happening to Bernie. It was not fair on her and I was thinking about what I could do to help her.

Then I had a brainwave about who could help me make sense of it all – my breast cancer nurse Sarah.

I peeled myself up from the hallway floor, dried my eyes and dialled her number.

'Bernie has breast cancer,' I blurted out when she answered the phone.

Calm and reassuring as always, Sarah expressed how sorry she was to hear that and asked which kind of breast cancer was it.

That flummoxed me.

'Oh, I don't know; I will have to find that all out.'

'Could it be a new cancer?' she asked me, and I said, 'Yes, it could. Would that be better?'

'Well, no cancer is good, Linda,' she explained, 'but I think it might be better if it was a new cancer, in the fact that they will treat it as a separate cancer on its own.'

That gave me a little bit of hope that all was not lost.

I then phoned Bernie. I told her how sorry I was and from the start she was very 'cancer – schmancer, I'm going to do this', and that positive energy never wavered.

During our telephone chat she told me she had looked it up on the internet – the thing they tell you not to do when you're diagnosed, but which everybody does anyway – and had changed her diet by going dairy- and sugar-free in a bid to try and help avoid the cancer spreading or coming back.

And then she asked me what chemo was like? I thought, ah, she may be living in London, miles away from me, but I can help her in that department.

I explained it all as best I could from my own experience and told her not to be frightened to ask for help, and that if she was feeling rubbish she would have a breast care nurse or Macmillan nurse to look after her, who she could call anytime.

She said the hardest part had been when she had to break the news to her beautiful daughter Erin who was only 13. Imagine having to sit your child down and tell her that news? My heart went out to her having to have that conversation with her young daughter.

Of course, Erin was scared that her mum was going to die, and Bernie did her best to explain the situation and reassure her, telling her, 'No, we're going to try and fight our best and I won't die.'

Before finding out she had breast cancer, she had planned a massive birthday party for her big 50th in London, and we were all meant to be going down for it.

However, she was told her mastectomy and reconstruction operation was booked four days before her birthday, so the party was hit on the head.

Myself, Maureen, my brother Brian, and his wife Annie travelled down to be there to support Bernie through her ordeal.

As she went in for her operation, I took Bernie's daughter into London to spoil and make a fuss of her. Erin and I stayed in this swanky hotel in Kensington, and we went to a premiere of a film that Bernie had been invited to: *Legend of the Guardians*.

Erin needed a few hours of normality to take her mind off her mother being in hospital and that day out really helped lift her spirits and let her be a young carefree girl again.

After Bernie's surgery I waited until her husband Steve and Erin had seen her before going in to visit.

She was discharged from hospital on her 50th birthday. There was a bag attached to her body, which collected the excess fluid draining from her breast, and so I gave her this little pretty bag that I had used to put my old fluid bag inside after my mastectomy because it looked nicer than seeing the fluid sploshing about inside the pouch.

Annie and Brian surprised her on her birthday with a visit, and Steve cooked her a lovely meal at home, and she snuggled up with him and Erin.

It was a far cry from what she had planned to do, but all that mattered was that the operation had been a success, she was alive, and she was able to proceed with the next part of the treatment.

When she had recovered from surgery and was deemed fit to start, Bernie began her radiotherapy and chemotherapy.

Like me she had been worried about hair loss caused by the drugs.

When it was Maureen's hen do, Steve and Erin brought her up to Blackpool to attend it and they stayed at my house.

She called me upstairs when she was getting ready and said, 'Look, Lin!'

Bernie whipped her wig off to show me her bald head, which had a few little wisps of hair sticking out here and there like a baby's.

'I think I'm going to shave my head,' she said, rubbing her scalp with her hands.

'I don't like looking in the mirror when it's like this. I just feel I look like a sick person, you know, and I don't like feeling or looking like a sick person. I think I'll feel more in control if I get it shaved.'

I said to her, 'Then, Bernie, you have to do what feels right for you.'

She never wavered in her decision-making, did Bernie. Once she made her mind up about a decision, if she said she was going to do something she did it.

I had told her to use the cold cap before she started chemo-therapy and had explained to her how it had saved my own locks during treatment.

Bernie was delighted there was an option to save her hair, and told me she was going to try it, but when she looked into it further with her oncology team, she couldn't bear that it involved being stuck on the ward an extra two hours on top of the several hours you were already spending there for your treatment.

Also, when they initially place the cold cap on your head, it feels like your brain is freezing. The uncomfortable sensation only lasts a few minutes and then you acclimatise to it, but it is not easy to stand that level of cold, and a lot of people find it extremely off-putting, Bernie being one of them. So, she chose to put up with having a bald pate.

I was so proud of how she had handled everything thrown at her; even when struggling with the horrific side effects of her Herceptin treatment, she kept going, never complaining.

It caused her mouth to break out in a cluster of ulcers. There must have been about 20 of them like open wounds. It was dangerous because she had stopped eating and she went into hospital, where they had to liquidise her foods. They had wanted to keep her in to carry on treating her until things calmed down in her body, but it was Anne's grandchild Ryder's christening and Bernie was his godmother.

She told the hospital, no, I'm not staying because it's my great-nephew's christening, and I need to be there.

She also had terrible blisters on her heels, which were agony to walk on, but even in all that pain she still made it up to Blackpool.

The morning of the christening I had to bandage her feet to give her some padding so they wouldn't hurt so much when she was in the church doing her godmotherly duties.

There was a small party afterwards at the local pub and she sat down, and went, 'I want a vodka and ginger ale, please.'

Here's me thinking she would take it easy with her mouth being in such pain, but she was having none of it and said, 'It already hurts so I may as well add vodka!' She was fun and there was never a 'poor me' from her.

Bernie just got on with it and then things really started to look up.

They told her that they had got the cancer and there was no sign the disease had spread.

Happy days and we could all finally relax – Bernie had beaten cancer.

One afternoon I took a call from her and as we chatted about this and that she revealed she was going back on the road for the UK tour of *Chicago*. She asked if I could accompany her in place of Steve because he had to stay at home to take Erin to school.

There was no question of me not going and supporting my sister, and I jumped at the chance.

It was like a mini adventure as we went first to Worcester then Wales followed by a trip to Belfast.

We were away for about three weeks in total, and while we were doing the show in Belfast, it was her 51st birthday.

Steve and Erin came across and surprised her, which was lovely.

She also had a big party in January 2012, with a 16-piece swing band, called the 'I kicked cancer's butt' party.

About 200 people came and it was held in a lovely hotel in Weybridge.

That's how she was. She was just fabulous – a warrior who did things her way.

When her hair grew back, she went straight out and had it dyed platinum.

'Bernie, you know you're not supposed to dye your hair after chemotherapy,' I chastised, 'you're meant to wait a little while.'

'Oh Linda, who cares? Who is going to hit me?' she teased back. 'It's a bit of hair dye. It's not going to hurt me, it's going to help me.'

Now I'm going to take a leaf out of Bernie's book and when my hair has grown back after chemo, I will dye mine platinum in her honour! The last time I lost and regrew my hair it came in grey like a Brillo pad, so it's getting the Bernie dye job the next time.

With that, life seemed to go back to normal for all of us, and Bernie was non-stop busy with work.

She called me one night in late summer all excited.

'Linda, the *Chicago* tour is going abroad to Europe soon – Monte Carlo! Do I go?'

'Hell yeah,' I replied. 'You're cancer free and Monaco is fabulous – GO! Take Steve with you.'

She took my advice, and it was arranged for me to travel down south to look after Erin at their home while they were abroad for the week.

It was great news and I think I was more excited for their sojourn to Monaco than they were. Things were looking up and Bernie had a bright future once more – or so I thought.

A few days before travelling Bernie called me to say she had found another lump, this time on her breast in the middle of her chest.

She said you could even see a slight outline of the bump on her breastbone pushing through the skin and she had been to see her breast surgeon, who told her he didn't think it was likely to be anything major but wanted to 'whip it out' anyway.

She was booked in for surgery two days after her return to England and, with that, she and Steve went off to Monte Carlo where they had a lovely time by all accounts.

Two days before she was due back, I took a call at her house.

It was from the cancer surgeon's secretary. They asked to speak to Bernie, and I explained she was away performing, but would be back in two days.

I initially thought that they were calling to confirm the operation date with Bernie, but the surgeon's secretary told me it was a matter of urgency that they spoke to her as soon as she returned to the UK.

Replacing the phone receiver down, I thought, 'Oh God, that doesn't bode well'. A feeling of anxiety took hold of me that I couldn't shake off.

I toyed with calling her in Monte Carlo, but I did not want to ruin her trip when I didn't know what the call was about, and she couldn't do anything from over there anyway, so I waited the 48 hours until she was back.

When Bernie arrived home, the first message that I gave her was that she was to call the hospital.

'Did they give any idea what it was about?' she asked, before going off to call them.

After dinner, when Erin had gone to bed, we sat in the lounge and she said the doctor had told her he could not do the surgery to remove the lump because the cancer had spread, and she was ordered to go in the next day for scans and tests.

'God, Lin, what if I go in and he says it's spread all over?' Bernie said, looking at me, her face full of fear. 'What if it's in my liver or my kidneys and what if he says it's in my brain – oh God, I couldn't bear that.'

It was understandable how frightened and worried she was, but I reassured her it was going to be okay.

She looked great, had been feeling great, and I told myself this would just be another blip and they would get on top of it again like they had with her cancer first time around and we had to be strong, even if we were all scared to death.

'Oh, don't be ridiculous, Bernie; you're just jumping the gun here. You have a little lump in your chest, and it's spread a bit further. So that doesn't mean the cancer is going to be all over. You may have to have a little bit more treatment to get rid of the lump there and it'll be fine again, come on.'

The following morning, Bernie went off with Steve to the oncologist and I stayed home to be with Erin, and she said they would phone me as soon as she came out of the hospital.

By 1pm I had not heard from her. She was seeing the oncologist at 11am and I knew from my own experience it didn't take that long to get your results.

No news is good news, I was telling myself, and maybe there has been a delay in the clinic with patients and she'll call any minute.

And then two o'clock came and she still hadn't phoned me. As each hour passed, I thought, oh my God, please let her be okay, and I just left a message saying, Bernie, please just phone me back and let me know how you got on.

By 4pm she called up.

'It's not good news, Lin,' she cried. 'It's spread and it's in my brain.'

That part destroyed me because she had voiced her concern about it going into her brain and I had dismissed that fear with a, 'Oh, don't be ridiculous.' I felt terrible and wanted to throw up, but I needed to get a grip.

What good would it do Bernie to have me crying and wailing?

Now more than ever she needed all of us in the family to be strong and together.

I vowed to myself that I would not let her down.

'Well, we can just fight it. You know, we'll fight it together,' I promised her.

Bernie explained the doctor had told her the cancer was treatable, but not curable.

'Yeah, but they haven't said it's terminal, have they, or given you three months?' I rattled on with various well-meaning platitudes to bolster her spirits. 'They can treat it, that's a great sign.'

I then asked if she was going to come home anytime soon, but she said she was going to sit a little longer in the hospital garden.

I understood she and Steve needed a place of quiet repose to take it all in.

'What do you want me to do? Do you want me to call the others in the family and tell them?' I asked.

'Yeah, if you don't mind. I can't face it.'

When she hung up the phone, I collapsed on the floor and sobbed my heart out.

Better to get it out my system so I was calm before I phoned the others because they were all waiting on tenterhooks for news.

'Hi Mo, I'm afraid to say it's not good news for Bernie.'

'Oh my God,' Maureen gasped.

'It's spread and it's in her brain and it's treatable, not curable.'

Then another voice came on the call and went, 'What's wrong? What's happened? Maureen's on the floor!'

It was Madison, Maureen's daughter-in-law, who told me Maureen had collapsed on the floor with the shock. I told her the sad news and she said she was sorry and would look after her.

Next up I called up my brother Brian to tell him, but I got no response. I left him a message asking him to give me a call when he got it.

'Oh no,' I thought, when I ended the call to his voicemail; he's a salesman and he's out working, and I shouldn't have left that message when he's on the road.

So, I phoned his wife Annie instead and asked for her to tell him when he got home.

Just as I finished speaking with her, Brian rang back.

'Hi Lin, how did she get on?'

'Oh, Brian, I was going to wait until Bernie came home from the hospital and then tell everybody together,' I said, doing my best 'not a care in the world' voice, hoping that would stall him until he was back home with Annie there to support him.

But Brian was not buying my brush-off and repeated his question, 'How did she get on?

He knew me too well and it was no use lying to him.

I told him and he was distraught. I'd never heard my brother this upset and had feared how hard it would hit him.

'Where are you?' I asked.

'Sainsbury's car park.'

Afterwards, he told me he sat in the supermarket car park and cried for an hour but that nobody knocked on the car window and asked if he was okay or needed help.

Poor man, I felt so sorry for him. He phoned his wife and she talked to him all the way home, so he had some moral support and comfort on the drive back.

My oldest brother Tommy then called me up to ask what he could do.

'Well, I think everybody's gathering at Maureen's house at the moment', and then just after he hung up the phone rang again.

It was Anne this time: 'Linda, what should I do?'

'Anne,' I said, 'I think you need to go around to Maureen's, please. She is with Madison, but she needs one of us there; she's in bits.'

Then I called Denise, who at that time was living in London, and she said, 'Well, when Bernie gets in let us know and we'll come over.'

A close friend of all of ours called Mark Rattray phoned me and I told him, and he got in the car from Coventry and just drove for four hours to be there for Bernie, which was amazing.

When Bernie got back to the house later that afternoon, I hugged her so hard, and we couldn't help it, we both cried.

Denise and her partner came over and Steve asked Bernie, 'What do you want to do Bernie, stay here or go up north with Linda?'

'I want to go back to Blackpool. I want to be with the family,' she said.

The next morning, we loaded the car and drove up. Bernie had chosen to stay with Brian and Annie at their house.

My late husband Brian used to call us Nolans 'the cavalry', and by the time we got there, it looked like they had all come riding into town. There were brothers and sisters who had all brought their partners with them, so there was a lot of hugging and then a lot of laughter and a bit of sadness, but more laughter than anything else.

We're Nolans, so that's how it is.

Bernie even had a cheeky vodka as we united around her, clucking like mother hens and fussing, in between asking each other, what are we going to do?

Sat in the corner next to Anne, I said, 'I haven't got a thirteen-year-old child who needs me and a husband. It's not fair on Bernie; it should have been me not her who is going through this.'

'It shouldn't be you,' Anne said. 'It should be me because I'm the oldest girl, but we can't talk like that, Linda – illness doesn't happen like that.'

We were all getting irrational by that point.

Bernie stayed in Blackpool for a week. None of us wanted to let her go but they had to return south so she could start radiotherapy treatment and for Erin to go back to school.

Radiotherapy is not pleasant but the way they do it on brain tumour patients is horrendous, because they measure your head and take a mould of your face and head and then this is made into a mask, which goes over you as you are having the treatment.

It's so awful an experience that Bernie had to be sedated to have it.

Throughout her months of treatment, we travelled up and down from Blackpool to Surrey each weekend to support her and Steve and Erin.

On one of those visits, Bernie confided to me she was arranging a surprise birthday party for her husband, in February.

She said his birthday coincided with the weekend she was coming to Blackpool on 21 February, where all our family were and a lot of Steve's friends from years back when they lived in Blackpool where they first met.

'I'm going to get four or five relatives in the north east where he's from to come down for it. Will you help me to organise it, Linda, because I'm in London?' she asked me.

'Yeah, it's the least thing I can do for you, just tell me what you want, Bernie.'

The next few weeks was full on as I organised everything – booked the restaurant she wanted in Blackpool, arranged balloons on the tables and decorations with a party planner and sent out invitations for everybody.

The venue looked fantastic and we all had our best party dresses on. I wanted Bernie to be happy and I was waiting for them at the top of the stairs as they came through the door.

She had all her make-up done and she looked gorgeous – stunning. But as she walked her legs went and collapsed beneath her, and there was a kerfuffle as everybody rushed to help her up.

'I'm all right,' she insisted, downplaying it, as she managed to get up. Steve, of course, was overwhelmed when he saw all the people waiting in the room for him – all his own family and friends from over the years.

Bernie was also delighted by his reaction and overcome too by the emotion of it all. I saw her eyes fill with tears.

I went across and asked her, 'What happened? Are you okay?', and she said, 'It was so weird, Lin, my legs just gave way, but I feel fine, don't worry.'

'Come on, then, sit down here and get yourself settled,' and I went and got a chair for her. 'What do you want to drink, Bernie?'

'Vodka!'

'Would you not like some water instead, Bernie?' I dared to suggest.

'Vodka, thank you,' and I knew better than to argue with her.

You didn't come between Bernie and her vodka mules at a party! She was the ultimate party queen, and I took it as a good sign that she felt well enough to enjoy a drink.

Despite the rocky start with Bernie's collapse, we all had a great night, and it was lovely all being together again in happy circumstances.

Her husband was thrilled and then, on the 23rd, it was my own birthday.

I'd booked a meal for the family at a local Italian restaurant. Steve called me and said that Bernie hadn't had a great night's sleep and was a bit restless.

I phoned Bernie and told her, 'Honey, please don't feel obliged to come to my party; go back to bed and just rest up.'

'No, I want to, but I won't have my make-up done and I can't stay late.'

She came to the party and you could tell she wasn't feeling great. We all love this restaurant – it's immaculate and none of us has ever had a bad meal there in all the years we've been going – but all of a sudden, she was moaning about the food, saying, 'This doesn't taste right.'

Bernie wasn't herself that night; it was clear she was not well at all. They left early, and on Sunday we got a phone call to say she had gone to the hospital in the night, because her breathing was really bad, but was out again.

My brothers, Steve and some other male friends had gone to the local pub for a lunchtime drink and we went round to see Bernie, where we found her lying on the couch. When I saw her, I had a flashback of my husband the night he was taken into hospital and I knew she was deteriorating rapidly.

'I don't feel great,' she said listlessly and started coughing. Once her coughing started, she couldn't stop to catch her breath. It was scary to witness.

'I'm calling an ambulance, Bernie,' I said, recalling that scene with Brian just a few years earlier.

'No, Steve, get Steve, please,' she begged.

I panicked when Steve wasn't answering his phone and so I quickly ran to the pub along the street to find them, and they all ran back with me.

When he saw her, Steve rushed to her side: 'There isn't time to wait for an ambulance,' he said, as he scooped her up in his arms and carried her outside to the car. He rushed her into accident and emergency, where they deemed her 'very poorly' and took her up to the cancer ward to treat her.

I phoned my breast cancer care nurse Sarah, who went around to see her on the ward, and she told me the palliative care team had already been there dealing with it and given Bernie some methadone to stop the cough and make her comfortable.

Thankfully, that meant Bernie was able to get some sleep.

But she added ominously that when the cough came back it would be towards the end.

My heart broke in two as I realised what was being conveyed between the lines – that there was no medical treatment to prolong her life, only to make her comfortable.

Erin was staying at my house with me, and Steve and Bernie, as any parents would do, were trying to shield her from the full extent of it until they knew more about Bernie's prognosis.

Despite knowing palliative care were now involved, I kept telling myself that Bernie was tough and would rally round. Positive thinking.

The next morning Steve called me from the hospital and asked if I would bring Erin in.

'Yeah, of course,' I said, trying not to think the worst.

'But when she gets there, Lin, will you get the nurse to bring her around, please? We just want to talk to her first.'

'Yes, whatever you need me to do,' I replied to him, and went back upstairs to tell Erin to get ready.

'Was that Dad on the phone?' asked Erin. 'How's Mum? Can I go and see her yet?'

I told her the coughing had stopped so her mum had managed to get some sleep and that she was looking forward to seeing Erin.

When we arrived, a nurse came and took Erin away as requested over to Bernie's room while I waited in the lounge.

After 15 minutes or so the nurse came into the waiting room and said: 'Do you want to come in?'

The scene in that hospital room is one I will never forget. Bernie was in the bed. Erin was lying beside her mum, holding her, and Steve was sitting on the chair beside them with his arms around both his girls like he never wanted to let go.

He looked weary and his face wore a look of despair that I recognised from my own face when I was told the news that Brian was going to die.

Bernie looked up at me and said, 'I'm not going to make it, Lin.'

'What do you mean?' My voice cracked with emotion.

'They told me this morning I've got two weeks at the most and I'm not going to make it. I'm not going to see my lovely house again.'

'We will make sure you get back to your lovely house,' I told her.

And just like when we had found out the cancer had spread, just three months earlier, Bernie asked me: 'Will you let the others know for me? I haven't the energy.'

'Of course, my darling,' and I went and kissed her, and then left them to be in peace together.

When I got outside the room, I started to cry, and this lovely nurse took a few minutes to stand with me and comfort me.

She reminded me of my sister-in-law, Annie, who works in the hospital. I called her and cried, 'Can you come down?', so she raced down and then we told the rest of the family.

It was decided that Bernie was to move to our local hospice, Trinity Hospice. The team there were fabulous and when she arrived its doctor said, 'Bernie, I want you to tell us what you want us to do for you.'

And she said, 'I want to go home.'

God bless her. They were marvellous with her and said, 'Okay, well, we'll make sure this happens.'

She had a lovely room at Trinity during her time there. There were two beds in the room so Steve could stay every night. They turned the bed around and they'd watch a movie on the TV as a family.

It was Mother's Day while she was in there, and we asked the hospice if it was okay for all of us to come down with a picnic for her.

They were fine about it, so we all arrived with treats and bundles of flowers. Erin had a present for her too, and it was a glorious day full of joy despite the circumstances.

Bernie was bright-eyed and looked beautiful. She had a big cheery smile for everybody; despite her being in pain with bedsores, I never heard her complain.

I hate to use the B word, but she was so brave. It would have been so easy to say, I'm not going out, or, I can't do this or that, but during the whole time she dealt with cancer she would never entertain any thought of giving up. Even when she became very poorly, she insisted on joining us on shopping trips.

Relatives from Ireland came over to see her, as well as friends from all corners of the UK, as they knew the situation.

The hospice told them they could use the day room, and Steve joked that, 'It looked like My Big Fat Gypsy Hospice', after the TV show *My Big Fat Gypsy Wedding* about the travelling community.

Brian accepted it, and that if you married one you married us all, and, as families go, the Nolans are solid.

There was that many people coming and going, it was amazing, and I was really pleased for her.

When we were sat around, Bernie said to us, 'You know, girls, I don't want loads of crying.'

Tommy, Denise and I excused ourselves and went outside to the nurse to cry because we didn't want to cry in front of Bernie. We did once or twice and she was fine about it but we tried to be strong in front of her.

Despite what was happening, Bernie stayed so strong and positive.

In total she was in the hospice for three weeks, living past the doctor's prognosis with the most exemplary care. Nobody could have cared or done any more than what she received in that brilliant place and they granted her final wish, which was to be at home.

The ambulance came and drove her all that way back to her beautiful home in Surrey.

Maureen drove their car back, following them down the road so Steve and Erin could hold Bernie's hands in the ambulance. She was delighted to be home.

There was an unpleasant incident during Bernie's last few weeks with us.

While we were in the hospice, Steve got a phone call to say the house had been broken into and the scumbags had stolen the TV and laptop and the car she was going to give to Erin.

When we waved Bernie off outside the hospice, we were all crying and there was a collective feeling that this might be the last time we'd see her alive.

When the ambulance turned that corner, I felt horrendous.

I don't think any of us knew what to think, what to say or do, or whether to go home. As a result, for an hour or so afterwards we just sort of stood around, crying and trying to pull ourselves together.

Meanwhile, when Bernie got home, bless her heart, she rallied again and even though we knew the results and what the outcome was to be, we almost started to feel hope that she could keep going as she defied the doctor's predictions and from being written off in March, she was still alive three months later.

During her time fighting cancer, she had written her life story. Steve had written the last chapter for her, and a television morning show asked him to go on and talk about the book when it was released on behalf of Bernie.

Maureen called me and said, 'Bernie wants you to come down today and stay with her as Steve is going to have to stay in a hotel before his TV appearance and I have to go to work.'

I mentioned Denise, who was nearby, and her other friends who had been going every day, and Maureen said: 'Lin, she wants *you* to sit with her.'

I was so thrilled Bernie had asked for me and was on the train to London two hours later.

Steve picked me up the other end from the station and said thanks so much for doing this, and I said, 'Oh God, don't be silly. It's fine, you know, it's me.'

He left about three in the morning; in the end the show had sent a car to pick him up and take him to Manchester, so he didn't have to stay away in a hotel.

I will say he was amazing at caring for Bernie. She wouldn't let anybody else do anything for her, even though we were all there and offering to do help, it was always, 'No, I want Steve to do it.'

He never got tired and nothing was too much trouble. He was her rock.

Before leaving, he went through administering Bernie's morphine into syringes and left instructions for me to help with managing her pain.

When it came to preparing the pain relief syringes, he'd measured them all out exactly with a strict timetable of what time her morphine was to be given, how to administer it and all the instructions/rota for the day until he got home.

When I woke up, I got up, put my dressing gown on and padded through to Bernie's bedroom, where she was already awake, waiting for her morphine.

She said she was feeling some pain and I quickly grabbed the morphine, but because it had been there overnight it was a bit sticky.

Steve had explained I had to be firm when inserting the syringe, so I pushed it like he had shown me, but it kept sticking and wasn't going in. I was nervous that I was hurting her, but typical Bernie, who was getting more exasperated by the minute, said, 'Just push it really hard!'

So that's what I did, and I think I almost killed her on the spot!

She went, 'Jesus Christ, Lin!'

'It got stuck!' I yelled, and we both started laughing.

Bernie sorted, I got Erin up, fed, watered, off to school, and asked Bernie if she would like to go back to sleep while I tidied up around the house and got the breakfast dishes washed.

Patting the mattress, she went to me, 'Come and lie on the bed with me, Lin.'

I went across and lay on top of the duvet and she took hold of my hands, and said: 'We've had a great life, haven't we?'

'Oh God, yeah,' I replied, thinking through our many wild adventures.

'It's strange, isn't it?' she said.

I knew she was referring to the knowledge her cancer was terminal, so I said, 'It's awful. You know, we all feel helpless we can't do stuff for you.'

'It's fine.' She sighed. She continued to hold my hands. 'Let's go to sleep, Lin.' And so we both fell asleep on the bed, holding hands like we were very young girls again.

It was lovely for me to share that precious moment with her – just the two of us with no distractions – and I wanted to soak up as much as I could of her while she was still physically present in our lives.

Later that day we had a visitor. Sally, our make-up girl from our reunion tour, had become very close to us all. When Bernie's house had been broken into while she was in the hospice in Blackpool, Steve's watch was among the things that had been stolen.

Bernie had had that watch engraved for his wedding present with some lyrics from their special song, and she'd taken advantage of Steve being out the way and asked Sally to come around with her laptop to help search for the same model of watch and arrange for it to be engraved, so she could give it to Steve as a special present.

A few weekends later, Maureen, Brian, Annie and I drove down for the weekend to see them, and we got there a little bit late because of bad traffic. We came in to find Bernie sitting in the lounge and Steve in the garden.

Bernie looked pale and very tired, but her face lit up on seeing us.

'Come on,' she said, beckoning us over, 'let's go out into the garden to see Steve.'

And so, we sat outside chatting happily and for a few minutes as we bathed in the prism of the sunlight, hearing her peals of laughter, it didn't seem real that Bernie was dying.

I could almost pretend everything in the world was normal.

Then the sun went behind a cloud causing Bernie to shiver and she wanted to go back inside the house to warm up.

I helped her inside and asked if she wanted me to get her a cup of tea and take her up to bed for a lie-down. Shaking her head, she motioned for me to sit beside her on the sofa and took my hand in hers.

'I've done you all proud, haven't I?'

I must have looked confused because, before I had the chance to answer, she carried on: 'You know, when they gave me two weeks. Well, I've lasted three months, haven't I?'

She really was incredible and it shows the power of the spirit and her sheer determination to keep going.

'Yeah, and that's brilliant,' I told her, blinking back the tears forming in my eyes. 'We've made some precious memories.'

'Linda, I need to tell you something. When I go, I want Steve to have this ring and I want Erin to have this ring,' she told me, twisting the precious metal bands off her fingers to show me.

I nodded that I understood and then she said to me, 'Can you believe we're talking about me dying?'

She saw in my face I was getting upset and answered her own question with a, 'Let's not, we will go to the garden and see Steve.'

She wasn't asking for permission to go or anything like that, but I felt she was coming to peace with dying and telling me she had given us all another three months with her, but she was getting tired.

On the Saturday morning it was a beautiful day.

'What are we doing today, Bernie?' I asked her.

'We're going down to the cricket club to have breakfast.'

I chatted to her as she got ready and saw she had these terrible bedsores. They looked horrendous, but the nurses couldn't do anything about them because she couldn't lie on her stomach with her cancer being in the lungs as well, by this point.

As she got ready, she cried every time she moved with the pain of the sores, but she was amazing, and after she'd got herself dressed, we all trooped down to the cricket club with Erin and the family.

We ordered two jugs of Pimm's – Bernie had some too – as we were watching the cricket and me, Annie and Bernie were having lots of girly talks. And then we came back home, and Steve did a barbecue. Her energy was amazing.

On the Sunday we woke up and Bernie wanted to go with us for a walk to get some fresh air – she was using a wheelchair by then – but again, she was in pain.

'Well,' I said, 'I will stay in with you if you don't feel up to it.'

'I do want to go,' she told me. 'It just takes a lot to get ready.'

What I didn't know was that 12 of the cast from *Chicago* wanted to see her that day and had arranged with Steve to come around to surprise her when we were back from our walk in Richmond.

Bernie managed to get dressed but she slept in the car. As we pushed her chair, it was obvious that she was struggling with the pain of the sores as she kept moving around to try and get comfortable.

She told us she wanted to go home so we pushed her back to the car and home where she was settled in the conservatory and could look out at the beautiful garden.

'Oh my God,' Steve said to Maureen and me, 'they have already phoned me about three times, and I have missed their calls,' explaining about the cast visit.

'They're in the pub waiting to come around and they've brought guitars and that. Shall I say it's not a good time?'

We were both mortified at the thought of these lovely people coming out of their way to see their friend and waiting in a pub for news.

We told Steve: 'Oh God, they've come to sing. You have to let them in.'

When they walked into the house, they entered the room in a line, quietly singing 'All That Jazz' from *Chicago*. It was just like the movie – magical. We cried. Bernie woke up with all the commotion and although she wasn't well her face was overcome with emotion on seeing them and she started to cry.

It was such a beautiful moment, and it was testament to how popular Bernie was that the whole cast came to sing to her.

The actors stayed an hour or so playing songs, and Erin sang one too with them from *Toy Story*. It was just beautiful, beautiful moments being made that day and after they left that afternoon, we got ready to go back up to Blackpool.

We were all in bits saying goodbye to Bernie, and Steve came out with us to see us into the car and let us out the gate.

As we were going, we turned around to see Steve standing there crying as we drove away.

We felt terrible leaving him like that, and it was a quiet journey back to Blackpool as we reflected on Bernie and the precious time that we had all spent together.

We got home tired on the Sunday night and Monday rolled on uneventfully as Mondays do.

I wanted an early night, still tired from the weekend and drive back, and got into bed about nine.

Just as my head hit the pillow the telephone rang.

I sat back up and turned the light on to get the phone, expecting it to be Mo checking how I was after the weekend, but it was Steve.

'You need to come back,' he said when I answered. 'She hasn't got long.'

I flew back out of bed, got dressed in record time, threw some fresh clothes and my toiletries in a bag, called Maureen and we drove down.

When we got there, she was ill in bed. The palliative care nurses were already in the room with her and she'd been put on a morphine pump.

Not much later our brothers arrived from Blackpool with their partners, and Anne came with her two daughters and our Aunty Theresa. Coleen was there too. Denise was away working on a cruise ship.

We brought chairs up from the lounge to sit on. It was the year that Andy Murray won Wimbledon. Coleen was sitting beside Bernie on the bed and every time Murray got a winning shot in the final, she was whispering to her: 15/love to Murray; 30/love to Murray. And then we started singing some songs.

Bernie let it be known she was not impressed by our singing. She lifted her hand up and made a no sign with her finger as if to say no singing, you silly bitches, so we stopped.

Before we went to bed that night, even though it was in July, we decided to sing another song, this time with our brothers – the Christmas favourite, 'Have Yourself a Merry Little Christmas'. Steve got out a bottle of champagne and poured each of us a small glass. He put one beside Bernie on her bedside table and we all raised our glasses and toasted her.

We went to bed and in the night, my brothers and Maureen were all woken by Bernie crying. Their bedrooms were situated nearer to Bernie's bedroom than mine, and Maureen came to wake and tell me.

Erin and I have always had a close relationship and she would always stay with me when she was little.

Mo asked if I would go and get Erin up because she needed to see her mum.

I knocked on her door and gently woke her. 'Erin, your mom is really poorly and you need to go in to see her'.

She realised what this meant, and I gave her a cuddle.

We went into Bernie's bedroom and Steve looked like he hadn't slept a wink, but he talked to us as Bernie lay sleeping.

The room was starting to feel stifling from all of us being cooped up together in there for so long, so a couple of us asked the district nurses caring for Bernie how long they thought she may have left. They told us, 'Well, don't go far. It's not imminent, but don't go too far.'

It felt good to get outside and take a little walk to stretch our legs, breathe in some fresh air and make meaning of it all.

Nothing had changed when we got back, and we gathered around the bedside in silence just watching her sleeping peacefully.

Steve had been holding Bernie's hand and looking at it he went, 'Oh, I think it's going to be today, her fingers are turning blue. I remember when my mam died, her fingers started to do the same. It's where your organs are shutting down; her blood isn't being pumped around the body and that's why her hands are going blue.'

I jumped up. 'Should I go downstairs and get the others?'

'Yes, I think you better do,' he instructed.

Remembering the times Bernie used to say to us following her cancer diagnosis, 'I just don't want to die on my own. I don't want to be alone when I die,' I ran downstairs to round everyone back up to the bedroom.

Trying to be frivolous when talking about death, we would fire back at her, 'Yeah, some hope of that, love!'

We all gathered outside the bedroom and it was decided it would be better if we went in individually to say goodbye to her as she started drifting in and out of consciousness.

When it was my turn to go in to say goodbye, I pulled the chair right up beside the bed and gently laid my head down on her stomach as I talked to her, and she just moved her hand and rubbed my head.

It was just so beautiful that she knew I was there when I was talking to her.

I sat back up and as I did so Bernie then screamed out something in her sleep and looked distressed. The nurses who were waiting just outside by the door heard the noise and came back in the room. They went to work, upping the morphine to settle her and make her comfortable.

Everybody else was called to go back in, and by this time she was on the way to being in a coma. We sat around the bed and Erin sat on the bed beside her mum. Bernie's breathing was becoming shallower, then we heard her try to take in a deep breath when we stopped talking and then she did it again. Erin told her, 'It's okay, Mummy. Everyone is here; Daddy's here and we love you.' The two of them wrapped Bernie in their arms.

For the third time she drew another big breath, and that was it ... she had gone. You could just hear sobbing from around the room.

It was the 4th of July. The nurses had told us she would die two days earlier, but Bernie had defied their predictions just as she had defied the doctors, and she'd waited until Independence Day.

You can't tell our Bernie what to do, even in death, I thought to myself.

There is no other word to describe losing my baby sister other than horrendous. Even though you think you are prepared, because you know it's coming, you are never prepared for that level of heartbreak; it was so hard.

When the funeral directors came into the bedroom to retrieve Bernie's body and take her to the funeral parlour, they said, 'It's not very pretty, you don't need to see this', because they were to put her in a body bag to carry her downstairs to the hearse as the stretcher wouldn't make it around the curved staircase.

Everybody disappeared away into the kitchen because understandably they did not want that image of Bernie being carried out the house like that imprinted on their minds.

But I thought, no, this isn't right – we can't let her be on her own – so I stood by the bottom of the stairs and watched them slowly and gently lift her down and onto a stretcher.

As they got ready to push the stretcher with Bernie out of the house, it came to me that this was the last time she would ever cross its threshold, and I asked the funeral director: 'Will you take care of her, please?'

'Yeah, don't worry, she's in great hands.' And with that she was gone.

• • •

Her funeral wasn't until 17 July, which sounds a long time, but it was delayed because Bernie and Steve's daughter Kate had been stillborn some years previously, and Bernie had expressed that Kate's body was to be interred with hers.

This involved asking the Home Office for permission, which they granted, and she and Kate were reunited.

Bernie's funeral was amazing and so moving. Hundreds of people came.

She didn't want it in a church because she wasn't religious and Steve is an atheist, so they had it in the Grand Theatre in Blackpool, because that was her church – theatres and show business.

It was just beautiful with a massive headshot of Bernie up on the stage and our brother was the master of ceremonies. Bernie being Miss Organised had arranged her funeral and chosen what poem she wanted Erin to read.

Erin read it for her before she died and they had even rehearsed it so she could hear it.

She also sorted out her own funeral car, casket, and for the wake to be held at the hotel where she and Steve had had their wedding reception.

A sour taste came when the hotel charged a fortune for the room and I felt they were really taking advantage of our grief.

They were total bandits, and they wouldn't give special rates for people travelling from Ireland for the funeral.

We would have gone anywhere else, such was their terrible treatment, but it was what Bernie wanted and we had to respect her wishes.

A video of Bernie singing the great Broadway song 'How Could I Ever Know' from *The Secret Garden* at a concert she gave at the Manchester Opera House was played.

The lyrics are so hauntingly melancholic – *'How could I know I would have to leave you? ... How can I say go on without me? ... Forgive me, can you forgive me and hold me in your heart ...?'*

It was heartbreaking and tragic, and Bernie sang it so beautifully.

Her daughter Erin and Steve were amazing all through the funeral and kept their dignity.

Bernie would have been so proud of them.

Maureen read out a letter Bernie had written in which she said: 'I've had such a great life. I've met my musical heroes, Frank Sinatra, Stevie Wonder ... I'm just sorry I can't be around to be old and to grow old disgracefully, with all of you.' She spoke about her daughter and her husband. And then, repeating what she had told us in the hospice, 'I expect tears but not lots of tears. I deserve a few tears but when you think of me please smile and maybe on my birthday, remember me with a drink ... and make it vodka!'

On her birthday I always remind people to have a drink for Bernie, and people take pictures of themselves with vodka and ginger ale and lime, and post them all over Facebook.

It's a really lovely way to remember her.

On the actual anniversary of her death, a few of us get together and mark it in different ways.

I get together with my brother Brian and his family, Maureen too and our other brother, Tommy, but Anne and Denise prefer to be at home with their own thoughts.

Months after Bernie died, there were days I was still struggling with her loss and I would go to call her to tell her a bit of news thinking she was there with us, just living at her house in Weybridge, and dial half the number only to remember she was no longer there.

We used to say, 'Oh, what are we going to do?' and 'What would you do without her?', and at times it was hard to comprehend she was no longer here.

But because of all my counselling, I now think of Bernie and smile because I remember the amazing person she was and how much fun she brought to all our lives. A part of me obviously can't bear that she's not here; when we're all together, we always say we can't stand it that Bernie's not here with us. But I do look and smile now and remember the lovely times that we had with her.

I think about her when I'm struggling with my cancer in my dark days and how she would handle things.

I tell myself Bernie would say, 'Just get out there, you can do it', or be the one going, 'Come on, get out of bed, we're going out. We're going to the park. Come on, you can do this.' She was always very positive and uplifting and fought it to her last breath.

She'd also be saying what the others are saying, such as, 'What can I do for you? How can I help?', and because she'd been through it, she would have her own advice and tips for all the side effects that you encounter.

And other times I think, Bernie fought so hard and yet it got her in the end.

I remember a nurse sat beside me who said, 'Your cancer is treatable, but it's not curable.' And I said, 'That's what you told my dead sister.' I felt bad afterwards for snapping and saying that to her, but I was upset, and they understood.

The nurse said to me, 'Everybody's cancer is different. You know yourself that Bernie's cancer came back and when it did it pretty much kind of spread everywhere, but yours is contained in your hip, and your outlook is very positive.'

So, I hear all that, but it's still hard sometimes to not panic or worry. Even when Anne got her great results, everybody goes, 'Now you will have great news.' When Denise said to me recently, 'It's gone,' I corrected her with, 'No, it hasn't gone; it won't go.'

I knew she meant it hasn't spread, but it's still tough to take.

Anne initially said in an article that she felt guilty when her chemo was to get rid of her cancer and it has done that, while mine is palliative chemo, but that she's realised that she shouldn't feel guilty because it's not her fault, she didn't do anything. When I read it, I said to her, 'Oh my God, I'm thrilled when you've got good news. Don't ever not tell me anything because you think it's going to impact on me or that, I will be thinking, "Oh great, you're better and I'm going to be here suffering with it still", because I'm not; I'm absolutely thrilled for you.'

It's just sometimes the cancer gets to your head and you can't help having morbid thoughts. I call them my dark moments.

They come sometimes at night as I try to fall asleep and my mind will start contemplating what it's all about, or I'll be having a cup of tea and sit down on the sofa for five minutes of relaxation, and these questions creep into your head, which you have no answer for, such as I wonder if I'll be here at Christmas or how many more Christmases I have, or will I see my godson getting married next year?

These moments of existential thinking partly stem from how Bernie's cancer came back the second time and the rapid speed she started to go downhill.

One moment she's living it up in Monaco, the next she's being told she has cancer of the brain.

The speed of her deterioration scares me, so when I think about how many months until the next Christmas and whether I'll make it, or if I'll end up like Bernie did, then I have to remember my cancer is contained and talk myself back into the present.

It's practically invisible in my hip and I tell myself hopefully with chemo it will be kept at bay and I can just carry on. And I do hear Bernie going, 'Don't go down that road, Lin.'

She's right.

There were times, however, when Bernie did allow herself to feel upset and she would say to us all, 'I don't want to die because I want to be here to see Erin grow up.'

She and Steve had so many plans. They dreamt that when Erin left home, they would buy a lovely property in Nice, France, and end their days there. Of course, it all goes out the window when something like this happens. Bernie even bought a big house on a hilltop in Cornwall before she died, with eight bedrooms and seven bathrooms. The plan was for all of us to go down there at different times to see her – she paid for it all – and even though it didn't happen, the thought of it was her way of keeping strong and keeping hope.

My breast care nurse once said to me, 'Don't ever take away her hope because when you've got no hope, you've got nothing.' I have never forgotten that advice.

When Maureen turned 60, she had organised a birthday party in Florida. Bernie desperately wanted to go and was crying because she couldn't fly there because of her medicine. Denise and I suggested to her, 'Why don't you cruise over?' But her husband was standing beside her shaking his head as if to say she won't be able to do that.

That response really hurt me. I made sure when Bernie was out of earshot to tell him what my breast cancer nurse had told me: 'Don't take her hope away. We know it's possible she won't be able to do it, but she got excited about it, so you know, that's a good thing.'

Steve acknowledged my point that day, and that's why she went on and bought this house in Cornwall, I think, because she wanted something to aim for in the future.

At one point the pair of them were going to go away for ten days to have a beach holiday in Bali or something when she first got ill, and she paid £1,100 for holiday insurance. The price from the insurance company was extortionate because she had cancer.

In the end they didn't take the trip because she was frightened to be so far away from home in case she became really ill and would not be with her doctors.

But despite those setbacks, Bernie was one of these people that just kept looking for the future.

The one thing she did not do was a memory box. I tried to suggest it to her indirectly and as sensitively as I could, that it would be nice for Erin when she turned 18 or 21 or when she gets married. And she didn't kind of pick up on it, saying to me, 'No, I don't need to; I've written her a letter.'

But when she was in the Blackpool hospice, she bought us all bracelets engraved with 'miracles can happen'. And with it were individual cards saying thanks for looking after me and I love you so much. It was just so amazing that she'd even thought to do that.

I think I'll do a memory box for the little ones if my cancer spreads further from my liver. One with a nice photo of me with everyone individually, my sisters as well as my brothers.

I'll have it framed so they'll have that when I've gone because I think I'm probably going to go before all of them.

And then of course, somebody might say, well, you might be here after all of them, because we've got a friend who has just celebrated her 80th birthday. She's had cancer five times! To that I'll say, okay, well, I want to be in your gang!

I do realise you have to get back to a normal life because otherwise you are just living cancer and that's taking the life you have away.

ANNE

When people ask me what was Bernie like, I tell them 'happy', because every time I saw her, she was always jolly.

I've thousands of special memories of Bernie.

I remember she was so fantastic right to the very end. She was amazing, always, no matter what life threw at her – that was Bernie. Her character didn't change, even when she got cancer. She was always positive. She would say things like, I'm going to beat this effing cancer and even towards the end, as she was walking around with an oxygen tank on, I never saw her moan or go 'why me?'.

During my daughter Alex's wedding, we were all together around the table chatting about the ceremony and she suddenly went, 'I'll never see my daughter walking down the aisle.'

She never usually said stuff like that or got melancholy or sad about it – she was always upbeat – and to hear her say that about Erin, who was only 12 then, was heartbreaking and we were all crying at the table.

One late spring afternoon, following a family lunch, we were sitting in her back garden playing a boardgame and we were being very sensitive to her and thought she wouldn't want to play as she was tired and had the oxygen tank, but being Bernie, she said, 'No, I want to play', and so she played for a while and we were having a lovely time laughing away.

I didn't know it back then but that was the last time I saw her alive. Bernie losing her life to cancer was horrendous and even now I still cannot believe she's gone. She was so vital and funny and fun.

My favourite childhood memory of her was from her being on stage. From the time Bernie could talk, she sang on stage with us. When she was two, she used to sing a song called 'Strollin'' by Flanagan & Allen. When they performed the song, they used to wear cloth caps and so Bernie would get up on stage, cloth cap on, and put on a Cockney accent. It was incredible to see this little girl with the big voice taking on these songs. It was all in working men's clubs mainly when she performed it, but I remember when she was about five, she sang at the Grosvenor House Hotel for the Showmen's Guild. It was packed and she walked around this massive dance floor, singing away. Well, the crowd went absolutely mad and lifted her up and carried her up around the whole audience who all gave her money and she ended up with hundreds of pounds!

From when she was little, Bernie was always good and an easy kid to get on with. I can't remember her crying or being naughty. She was very inquisitive as well, a bit like Linda is, but I think she was shyer than Linda. She was not as extrovert when she was a tiny child as Linda was.

Her diagnosis was a tremendous shock to me, and my whole family, and it brought my own battle with cancer from ten years earlier flooding back into my mind. The anxiety was terrible and while you learn to live with it, it's always there at the back of your mind whether your cancer will return, just as Bernie's did.

So, because of this I don't like to dwell on it too much. I don't like to talk about it. I don't like to think like that, so perhaps my brain blocks it out and I blocked out an awful lot of her illness.

I remember her having a mastectomy. I remember her cancer, but I don't remember dates and times and what I was actually doing at the time. And maybe that's my brain's way of dealing with it, you know, not dwelling on it too much.

Thank God Bernie and I made up and were reconciled long before she passed. Bernie said to me before she died that she wished our row had never happened and that she wanted me to go on the Nolans 30th anniversary tour – the very thing that caused our falling out as sisters in the first place.

I told her, 'We are not talking about that. It's done and over with.'

And it is.

When it was her 60th, we got in touch with Steve and Erin and told them, 'Thinking of you today' and Erin said, 'Yes, thank you so much. Love you too.'

I also speak to them at Christmas.

When Bernie was dying, I remember we all went up to her house and gathered around the bed to talk to her. She'd been given morphine and we were all talking to her and we actually sang what we always sing – an a cappella version of 'Have Yourself A Merry Little Christmas' because she was not going to make

Christmas. Her husband asked us to sing it at the end of the bed. And we all sang it, and we hope she heard us. I was staying with Denise and Tom at their house, so I went home with them that night. We got up early the next morning and were driving across to Bernie's and one of the girls phoned us and said, you need to hurry, she might not last till you get here, but unfortunately when we got there she had died. When we arrived, Steve said, everybody has been up individually to talk to her, do you want to go?

'Yes, please,' I said, 'I'd like to.'

I went up and obviously she was on the bed, and Linda was in the room. She asked me if I wanted her to go, and I said, if you just go for ten minutes, and so she left the room. I just lay across Bernie and I sobbed. I initially didn't even say anything to her. I put my head on her chest and put my arms around her neck and then I just sobbed and sobbed and told her I loved her.

I'd give anything to hug her, see her smile and hear her voice again.

CHAPTER 8

HIPS DON'T LIE

LINDA

After losing Bernie, I didn't spiral out of control like I had with Brian. My family and myself were united in our grief and supported each other through the process.

I also had the coping mechanisms from years of therapy and counselling so I could put those measures in place to stop me from going into free fall.

Life fell back into its usual patterns of work and family and friends over the next few years and there was nothing eventful to report.

I was having bi-annual scans and would be signed off every six months and it was all just a routine, everything's fine type of thing.

One night in 2017 I was babysitting my three great-nieces. I was walking up the stairs when I missed my footing and fell forward at the top. I heard a great big crack and couldn't move I was in so much pain.

All of the children were downstairs watching television and I was screaming their names millions of times. Sienna, five, and Ava, seven, eventually heard my cries and came out of the living room and looked up the stairs to see me lying there prostrate across the landing.

But bless them, because of their young age they thought I was just playing a game. Ava turned to Sienna and told her, 'Aunty Linda is pretending to cry.'

'No, I'm not messing about girls. Please come up here.'

They tentatively came up the stairs and, like an old woman, Ava went: 'Aunty Linda, whatever is the matter?'

'Please don't be frightened, Ava. I just need to get my sisters to come around so can you get my mobile phone? It's downstairs.'

I told them where they could find it and Sienna went to retrieve it while Ava stayed by my side.

Sienna came back with the phone and told me, 'Aunty Linda, I've unlocked the door for Mummy to come in and help you.'

I could have cried again at what a little pair of heroes they were. I called my brother first but he was engaged, then Denise, who called Anne to assist.

When I hung up, Sienna had these big fat tears coming down her cheeks and I said to her, 'Sienna, darling, please don't be sad. It's just like when you fall over in the playground and hurt your knee. The doctors are coming, and your mum is on her way too, so all is going to be fine.'

'Oh, it's not that which is upsetting me,' she declared crossly, something of a pet lip sticking out.

'What's it about then?' I asked, feeling a little miffed my current plight was no longer her number one concern.

Turns out Sienna wanted a sleepover and was upset this plan was all hit on the head due to my accident!

I had already called 999 for an ambulance; when they'd heard me scream from the pain, they had paramedics to me within an hour.

After examining me, they said something had cracked and took me into A&E. I thought I was finished with the bloody place and now I was heading back with what we suspected was a fracture to my leg.

The nurse sent me to X-ray, even though I told her it was not a big fall.

Turns out the crack that I'd heard on the top of the stairs when I smashed the ground was the top part of my hip bone snapping and it needed further investigating to find out what had caused such a deep fracture like that on a soft impact surface.

I was sent to the Orthopaedic Hospital in Oswestry, near Wales, which is a centre of excellence for bone cancers, and I was given a bone scan and biopsy. The consultant, called Mr Cool, was quite attractive and he kept calling me Linda when he was talking to me and I was thinking, how does he know my name when he has not looked at my notes? Is he a secret Nolans fan? But it turns out it was written on the noticeboard behind my bed – hilarious.

The biopsy was done through keyhole surgery, where they took a piece of the bone to test and it was done under general anaesthetic.

That's when I started to get upset. I was going through this again and didn't have Brian this time to be there to hold my hand.

I was miles away from home and I was so distressed that the nurse who had attended me in the recovery ward came to see me in my room before she went home.

Dr Cool came to see me two days later with the results and said, 'I think you know, Linda, there is cancer in your hip. But it has not extended; it has stayed localised.'

It had, by all accounts, been eating away at the bone where the hip meets the pelvis.

He reminded me to stay positive because my cancer was contained, and I had been cancer free for the best part of a decade.

I thought about Bernie and how her body had been riddled with it, and retorted, 'Yeah, but that's what you told my sis.'

To this day I still don't know how I tripped and fell up the stairs. The others joke it was Bernie pushing me, like some guardian angel causing a divine intervention, so my cancer was caught early.

Well, Bernie always pushed me in life, so why not in death too?

'I'm going to send you back to the north west to your oncology team there, where they will get in touch with arrangements for your radiotherapy,' Dr Cool announced.

It all moved fast and when I started treatment at the cancer centre in Preston, I walked in and thought, oh, nothing has changed in a decade.

They're a brilliant team but it did feel like being in *Groundhog Day* where I was back to getting my little voucher for free tea and biscuits and organising pick-up and drop-off times with family.

They all rallied around, offering to take me each day for my treatment, and Denise insisted I came to live with her and Tommy for a bit because she has a walk-in shower, which made life easier for me after my hip operation.

I did have a wallowing moment of feeling sorry for myself when I got a skin infection from the radiotherapy and was on antibiotics for weeks. But like the first time I had cancer I kept going and lived my life to the full in between quarterly scans, confident my cancer was being held at bay...

CHAPTER 9

FIGHT TO SURVIVE

ANNE

During the first UK lockdown, the weather was lovely and sunny, and I was lucky to have a garden to go and sit in and enjoy the spring sunshine and temperatures warming up.

I developed this routine, which was basically a continuation of holiday mode from just coming off the cruise liner. I'd get up, potter about, have a shower, some breakfast, get my book or download a podcast and spend late morning and lunchtime in the garden soaking up the lovely spring sunshine.

The day I found my new lump started like all the others had been in lockdown. I was in the shower washing myself as you do when I felt a lump under my left breast.

'That doesn't feel normal,' I told myself. I continued washing, wondering if I had chanced upon another cyst.

Jumping out the shower to dry off I searched again for it but couldn't find it. Maybe I just imagined it, I thought, and got dressed.

Later on, I remembered pressing on something that hadn't felt normal and started to think, was it really there or maybe it's gone because that's what you wanted. You want it not to be there.

I tried feeling about again and couldn't detect it so I switched off as I didn't even know if there was a lump definitely there to get upset about.

The next day when I was having a bath, the thought of the lump came back in my head, and I examined my breast again as I lay back relaxing in the hot water. I moved my hand around searching but still didn't feel anything. False alarm I thought but with my hand still on my breast I shifted position to move forward and sit up when, bang, there it was.

I continued to move my fingers over it, back and forth almost as though rolling it. It felt smooth, round and hard – like a marble and similar in size to one. It wasn't painful.

I lay back again, pressing my fingers around the area, only for it to vanish once more.

There was no denying it, something was there, and the fact it only appeared when I leaned forward didn't fill me with confidence either. I jumped out the bath to call the doctor and request an emergency appointment, and of course all the time I think, please don't let it become a lump; please just be a cyst that they can aspirate.

When I arrived at my GP surgery, it was like something from a science fiction movie – eerily quiet, staff in full PPE.

I tried to stay calm as my doctor examined me.

It was hard to read her thoughts as she moved her hand around and I explained how by chance I had come upon it.

'Okay, I'm going to send you to the breast care clinic just to check it's not nothing sinister,' she announced.

As soon as she said that I knew something was not right this time. I'd had loads of lumps, which she had aspirated before. Now she was telling me that I needed to go for a mammogram. I went home and I thought: it's going to be cancer.

As soon as I got home I called my daughters and sisters and told them about finding a lump and what had been said by the doctor.

I said to them, I think it's going to be bad news, and they started chastising and shouting at me, saying for, 'For goodness sake, have some optimism, would you, please?'

I replied: 'Well, there's no point in me having optimism because I know in my heart what it's going to be. And if I'm too optimistic and then he tells me you're doomed then I'm going to be devastated.'

Trying to do as they suggested, I also reminded myself that I had suffered lumpy breasts before my first brush with cancer – anything to stop the thought I had cancer again coming into my head.

My last mammogram was in 2017, which was clear, and I regularly checked for lumps so if it were something sinister it would be new and not have had time to have grown dangerously big, I told myself.

Our breast care clinic in Blackpool is fabulous and this is where I went for my mammogram and I was seen within the week, which was incredible given the scenes that we were starting to see about the pressure on our wonderful NHS staff and hospitals. Despite the pandemic raging, the service and care I got was always exemplary.

As well as having a mammogram, a needle biopsy was carried out to extract cells and tissue sample for testing. During the wait to speak to the surgeon, I thought: it's cancer. They know it's cancer and they're not telling me they know where it is because they wouldn't be doing all this to me.

The surgeon said to me that from observing the mammogram results alone: 'I'm ninety-five per cent sure it's cancer, but obviously I'm not infallible and you should wait for the results to make it a hundred per cent.'

What choice did I have other than to say, 'Okay, fine?' But I decided to try and live on the 5% hope he had given me in the meantime.

That week at home was excruciating, having to wait for confirmation, but once back in the surgeon's office he said the results of the biopsy showed it to be another grade three tumour like I'd had the first time 20 years ago.

I didn't sit back in shock this time when he confirmed it was malignant because I had already resigned myself to it being cancerous, but I did sit wondering when it could have appeared, and my mind started rewinding year by year.

After my first all-clear from cancer in 2005, I was having scans every six months then down to annually and then every three years in line with the national average, as screening is still the best form of cancer detection.

On that premise, this new cancerous tumour should have been picked up in 2018 and I was given a form to sign, saying I would like to have it investigated as to why it didn't detect it.

On the day it was announced this book was coming out I received a letter saying things couldn't be taken any further by the hospital, effectively saying it was not there and they did not miss it.

I suppose cancer can develop at any time, people are human, and errors do happen, and I think that's why we should offer annual mammograms like other countries do.

Fortunately, my cancer was contained, and I was referred to oncology for chemo.

Here we go again I thought when I went off to meet the oncologist.

He told me straight off I would be having chemotherapy, an operation, and radiotherapy to blast the bugger away for good. Then further treatment or Herceptin after that.

I wasn't looking forward to the chemotherapy because the first time round had been hard to take, and with this lump being a grade three, I knew the treatment would be a bit more aggressive and stronger.

Trying to be strong and positive I told myself you've been through it before and you can get through it again. Lying in bed alone at night is the worst part of the day I find when you live with cancer. Fear will set in as I am lying in the dark, alone, and I will panic, thinking, am I going to die? Will it be in two weeks or two years?

Another part of anxiety around this cancer was trying to deal with it under the burden of the pandemic.

I was so scared of leaving the house. I was even scared of taking things like letters. I was spraying everything that came through the doors with disinfectant.

When Maureen called to say Linda and I could have our chemotherapy treatment together, I cried with relief.

Knowing Linda and I have each other throughout this ordeal makes dealing with the tough burden of cancer that little bit easier to bear. We've shared every emotion – the highs and the lows – and we are stronger together because of it.

Two decades earlier when I had my chemo for the first time, I could go out and do things. I could go to the cinema and the theatre. I could go to restaurants. I could go and stay with my daughters overnight, if I wanted to, see my grandchildren, I could even go to work if I wanted to, you know, which I did.

But I couldn't do any of that now, because of all the lockdowns and restrictions, especially as I was having to shield when I was having chemo. It was horrendous.

The first thing they tell you when you have any cancer treatment is that it's very bad for you to get an infection. If you get Covid, there is a higher chance you can die because of what the treatments have done to your immune system. It's been like living in a nightmare really. And I know there's other people who are bedridden, who were actually in hospital the entire time having chemotherapy without any other family contact, and that made me think, I'm better off than a lot of people, you know; even though it's been a nightmare. It's been the worst thing I've ever been through in my whole life but I know there's people who've gone through worse.

Side effects of chemo aren't pleasant I must admit and sometimes a sense of humour is required to get you through it.

If you are squeamish you may wish to skip the next paragraph!

The reactions to my chemotherapy include constipation; and then I had diarrhoea really bad at one point. And then I had constipation again. So, I was taking medication for that as well. My poor intestines. It wasn't an experience I'm in a hurry to repeat.

I ended up not making the toilet once, which was really distressing. Remember that scene in the film *Bridesmaids* when the girls all have food poisoning in the wedding dress shop and there is a mad dash to the toilet, but the bride doesn't quite make it and she has to go in her wedding dress?

Fortunately for me I was home when it happened and not out and about like that!

Incontinence is another lovely side effect that no amount of pelvic floor exercises will remedy. I had to concede to it and ask Maureen to pick up some Tena Ladies protective pads for me to wear because I can't take the risk of incontinence striking me if I'm going to be out longer than an hour.

They are comfortable and I feel so much more confident walking around in case there are no toilets when it strikes.

These are things that people don't think about. The side effects of chemo are not just losing your hair; they are lots of other squeamish things like accidentally pooing yourself. Thank God it never happened again but you have to be able to joke about it to get through it.

On my third session of chemo, because I'd had those two reactions, I then started to get anxiety and racing thoughts of: I can't do this, it's too much.

And one day at the end of June I became gravely ill. My temperature soared to 38.8 and Maureen was there with me in the bedroom looking after me. I was freezing despite my temperature and the warm summer weather outside and I had to put a big fluffy hooded dressing gown on.

Maureen called the hospital for me and explained my reaction and it was suspected I had sepsis and I was rushed into hospital.

Hearing the word sepsis filled me with dread and I knew time wasn't on my side if I didn't get treatment fast. Sepsis or blood poisoning is a life-threatening infection that kills more people than heart attacks or cancer. The immune system goes into overdrive to an infection leading to poor blood flow and starts attacking your own tissues and organs and can kill in as little as 12 hours.

As a cancer patient undertaking chemotherapy my immune system had taken a hammering and I was ripe for infections to take hold in my body. My heart was racing from whatever was attacking me. My pulse rocketed up and they struggled to bring it down. It was terrifying thinking I could have a heart attack at any second and I wore a heart monitor for the next 24 hours.

The worse part was wondering what if I never see my beautiful family again? Due to the COVID restrictions even emergency patients weren't allowed family to visit and if I have sepsis then my chances of recovery are not really in my favour.

For nine days I lay there on my own with just the doctors and nurses for company being treated for suspected sepsis with intravenous antibiotics, trying not to think about what was to become of me and if I would ever walk out that hospital. My fears were also heightened by the thought of getting COVID on top of everything else I was going through. Everything felt bleak and I didn't want to die alone. It was one of the most frightening moments of my entire life.

After what seemed like an eternity - having blood tests every single day; my arm was so sore - they came back to me and said there was no sign of infection in my blood, and they suspected the symptoms were actual caused by the severe side effects of chemotherapy as opposed to a life threatening blood infection. And I think probably 50% of it was anxiety because anxiety can manifest itself physically and make your body feel ill.

The relief I didn't have sepsis was so strong I burst into tears. I could go home again and see my lovely children and grand-children. It was an experience I never want to go through again.

Every bad side effect chemo has the potential to cause – well I had them all. I got mouth ulcers like you've never seen. I couldn't taste anything; and even if I could taste it, I couldn't eat it because I was sick all the time. The doctors prescribed a medication to me to help curb the nausea and vomiting, but it didn't seem to really work on me very well. And even the times when I didn't feel sick, if I ate something, everything tasted off. And it wasn't just that I couldn't taste it; some of the food tasted absolutely awful. It was the same with the drinks – some drinks were okay, and other drinks not so good. I tended to have to keep drinking mainly water through my chemotherapy; there were times when even that tasted horrible.

Poor Maureen was cooking all these lovely meals and she would bring the food in and put it down, and I'd take one look at it, cry 'Oh God', and want to be sick.

She'd go, 'Come on now, Anne, it's not that bad.' I would feel mortified and have to explain, 'It's not your cooking, it's me!'

I felt terrible for her shunning all her lovely food she'd spend ages preparing to try and tempt me into eating something. I would also lose my voice when I got tired. And my eyesight's deteriorated rapidly, along with my hearing.

They give you loads of booklets to read before you start and sometimes, I think it's too much information to be bombarded with in one go. I don't want to know that much to start with; just let me get on with it and find my own coping mechanisms. But Maureen and I have read some of them as well, and they do say that in time things will return to what they were.

The worst aspect for me has been the constant feeling of pins and needles in my feet and hands, which Linda also suffers from. She has been amazing, trying to help me through it despite being run down by it herself.

It's called neuropathy and there is a warning it can last long-term, which I fear happening as it's dreadful. Truly it is horrible and drives you half mad.

When I was having all these side effects and an adverse reaction, I remember saying to my oncologist, Mr Bezecny: 'The bloody chemotherapy, it's killing me!'

He got upset and said indignantly, 'It will not be the chemo-therapy but the cancer that will kill you. Chemotherapy will save your life.'

And that's all you can pray for, that it does its job, which it's done. And that's fantastic.

LINDA

Cancer was the furthest thing from my mind when we got back to the UK from our cruise.

Although a lockdown was on its way, I didn't know then what was in store. I had a three-month tour to look forward to, which obviously got cancelled; Maureen was supposed to be doing a pantomime, also cancelled; and we, like the rest of the nation, followed the rules and stayed in our homes as Covid wreaked its path of destruction around the world.

When I got the call to tell me Anne had found a lump, I was lying in bed on a perfect spring morning, a Wednesday, thinking supermarket shop followed by walk or afternoon in the garden – so many endless options at that time …

It was Maureen. Just like when she told me about Bernie, she was the one to let me know about Anne.

Mo came straight to the point and said Anne had found something in her breast while showering and had had it looked at straight away, and the doctor said she had a breast tumour.

I was stunned. I think my face went white from the shock. It was the last news I was expecting. Covid went out of my mind and I thought, oh God, what can we do to help her? Can I be of assistance in any way?

And then things really went crazy. Just as I was coming to terms with Anne's devastating news, 30 minutes later my doctor's secretary from Blackpool Victoria Hospital called. With my cancer metastasising in my hip three years prior, I was given quarterly scans from my thorax down to my pelvis. I was told, 'Mr Danwata wants you to have an MRI scan because he saw something on your CT scan on your liver.'

If my heart was already jittery, it literally missed a beat during that call.

'Oh God.'

'Don't panic,' she said, 'because your liver has loads of blood vessels.'

I couldn't tell my family when we were dealing with Anne's diagnosis. I didn't dare say anything to anybody while I waited to have my MRI, and it was torture when the family were collectively saying how shit this was to have happened to Anne but, 'Look, Linda got through it a second time, and you'll get through it and all of that.'

I was staying at Maureen's house and after two or three days I thought I've got to tell someone because I can't bear it, so I said, 'Mo, I've got something to tell you.'

She went, 'What?' – she was peeling potatoes as I told her – and I told her my CT scan had shown something on my liver, and that they wanted me to have an MRI the following Monday.

She put the potato and knife down, and she said, 'Oh Jesus, are you joking?'

I said, 'Do I sound like I'm joking?'

'When did you hear?'

I told her three days ago, and that I hadn't told anyone else yet.

Mo looked hurt. 'You should have told us, Lin,' she said, giving me a massive hug.

But as I said to her, everybody was so sad and traumatised about Anne, I didn't want to make it worse.

Mo was great; we sat down to make a plan of action and she asked when I was going to tell the others. I said I wanted to wait another couple of days.

Mo and I used to take my dog for a walk about 6pm when the park was empty so we would stop on the street outside my brother's house on the way to the park and talk through the window.

He looked very upset when we got there and sighed. 'Poor Anne. God, I said to my boss, I just got over my sister Linda's cancer and now Anne's got it.'

Mo shot me a warning look and I whispered to her, 'I can't tell him now because he will be distraught – they've taken it bad about Anne.'

When we got home, Maureen brought it up again and told me that while I feel terrible now it might help Anne, knowing she's not in this alone.

'Okay, tell them now,' I told them.

She called them, and then they all phoned me, and said: 'We would be there in a heartbeat, but we can't because of Covid.'

Being told I had cancer during the pandemic and lockdown was much worse than previous times because they couldn't put their arms around me when I told them.

The following Monday, I went to have my MRI with my Macmillan support worker, which coincidentally was when Anne was having her first chemo at the hospital. As I got ready, my hands shook with nerves.

I had that feeling, like on your first day of school, or going to the dentist, which I'm scared of: one of total dread.

Maureen came with me and she was trying to do idle chit-chat, stuff like, isn't this a beautiful day, and telling me fun things about the kids to try and brighten everything up and keep me positive.

We got in her Honda and I was quiet on the journey. Staring at the road ahead, not knowing where my own future was taking me anymore, I said: 'What if it's back, Mo?'

'You know what? If he says it is cancer, we'll just get on with it, all of us, like we've always done. And you'll fight it, like you did the last time. And before you know it, you will beat it and be fine,' Mo replied.

That was my message of hope and I held on to that thought all the way to the hospital.

We parked up and made our way inside and, although it was one flight of stairs, we took the lift because my hip was sore.

Arriving at the ward I was greeted by the Macmillan nurse, who asked how I was. I told her I didn't know how I was because I hadn't spoken to Mr Danwata.

'You'll be fine,' she said cheerily, and went off to fetch Maureen and me a cup of tea.

After a short interval we were called through. There was a nurse in there as well. I introduced Maureen and we all stood around as though at a cocktail party making idle chit-chat for a few minutes, exchanging pleasantries about how things had been under the pandemic.

I first met Mr Danwata when he was the registrar in 2006 under his boss, Dr Susnerwala, who treated my cancer the first time.

Mr Danwata is a big believer in being mentally as well as physically fit. We patients all love him because he explains everything really clearly and shows pictures to make it all make sense, but the one thing that gets on my nerves is he goes 'be positive now', which makes me want to punch him and go, 'Mr Danwata, that's why I'm doing all this treatment,' but I would obviously never do that as he's lovely and I feel safe in his hands.

But back to the room, where I cut to the chase. 'The secretary says you've seen something on the CT scan?'

'Well, the MRI I asked you to have proved it is cancer. It's secondary. Again, it's spread from your breast to your hip, but now there is cancer in your liver as well.'

I just put my head in my hands as he delivered the rest of my sentence.

The good news was that he said of the mass of cells in the liver, 'It's very small, very tiny.'

'Please tell me I don't have to have chemo?' I sighed at him, still not lifting my head from out my hands.

And he told me exactly what I did not want to hear.

'Oh my God, it just gets worse and worse,' I wailed, not looking up.

'You know, there is a cold cap you can wear, which can help decrease hair shedding?' he said, as though I was a cancer novice.

I was severely pissed off by this point and stopped feigning politeness. This was the third time I'd had this wretched thing in my body so I cut to the chase and sharply retorted: 'So this is going to be how I live the rest of my life, Mr Danwata? You know, getting another cancer diagnosis year after year?'

I could feel the anger rising in me up to my throat and face.

Maureen had her hand on my back, trying to keep me calm, and I could hear her saying, 'You're going to do this. You've done it before.'

I just looked at her, and then I saw her crying, and the nurse gave us tissues.

Taking them, we walked out the room and sat in a little side ward for a few minutes to let me compose myself.

I wanted to run away from the hospital and get back into bed pretending none of this was actually happening to me, but I knew I needed to hear the rest and went back into his office. Mr Danwata kindly motioned me to sit back down and gently explained the cancer was not curable, which is depressing as they're just keeping it at bay until they can't really.

The whole thing was starting to feel surreal and I wanted it to be a bad dream I'd wake up from.

'How many cycles of drugs will I have?' I asked.

'The oncology unit will be in touch with you to start your chemo. I am suggesting you have six cycles every three weeks.'

He gave me the paperwork to take away with me, which had written on it 'palliative chemo'. I know that the cancer isn't curable but seeing it written down like that just makes it real, that it's just to buy me time.

It was awful and I got sad thinking about all the children – nieces, nephews, grandchildren – thinking, will I see them grow up?

And then I gave myself a good talking to.

Is this how you're going to be? Are you going to let yourself do this for the rest of your life, worry about what may be? Because if you do that then cancer has won. Do not let it destroy the life you have, which could be many, many years, or it could be a year or two years or six months, but don't let it destroy that.

And I felt empowered; this is something I will meet head on, I decided, and do as I did three years previously, which was give it everything I have.

It also makes you prioritise everything and value spending time with people that you love over everything.

And having gone through this THREE TIMES you've got to think like that, otherwise you spend every day depressed because you've got cancer. Cancer has won. But like in a boxing ring you've got to find the strength and courage to get back up and throw another jab at it.

Maureen put her arms around me, and Mr Danwata did his Mr Positive spiel, and when he finished talking, I told him, 'My sister Anne is going through it at the same time – she's in now having her first chemo session.'

Then it was his turn to be shocked. His eyes widened in surprise and he went, 'Oh boy, that's difficult.'

'Well,' I said, doing my classic trying to make light of the situation and be funny, 'maybe we could have our chemo together.'

To my astonishment he said, 'I will talk to your sister's consultant and see if Anne can go a couple of days sooner so you can be together for when your sessions start.'

I went to shake his hand to thank him, of course forgetting I wasn't allowed with Covid. He politely ignored my handshake and sat back down and told me: 'Remember Linda what I keep saying, being positive is as important as your drugs. You know your drugs can make you better. Keeping positive keeps your mind positive and this all helps. You've done it before and got great results and you will do it again.'

He was right of course. Having that positive belief that you will beat it was important, but sometimes you do just want to cry, and I think that's okay too because bottling up your emotions doesn't help in the long term. You've got to let it all out.

Maureen asked as we came out the hospital what I wanted to do.

'I'd like to see everyone.'

'Okay Lin, let's call Denise first and ask if we can all meet in her back garden where we can socially distance.'

As she was doing that, I phoned Coleen, who was waiting on news from her home in Cheshire.

'It's not good news Col, it's in my liver.'

Coleen took it as best she could and rallied behind me, saying how we would get through it again and the family were all behind me.

Denise handed me a large gin when I arrived at the garden gate, and the others had a cup of tea. I stayed that night with Maureen again.

When I was back at mine a few days later Maureen phoned me and said Anne is really up for having her chemo with you because she is so anxious about the whole thing and would love it if you could have your sessions together.

Mr Danwata was as good as his word and arranged it for 6 June.

CHAPTER 10

CHEMO SISTERS

LINDA

You have heard of the dance DJ group the Chemical Brothers; well, I named me and Anne the Chemo Sisters!

Our first chemo together was on 6 June. Tom and Denise dropped me at the hospital and, because of Covid rules, they couldn't come in with me or even just walk me to the door.

Denise cried, telling me it was because, 'It feels like leaving your four-year-old at the school gate; you'll just walk off with your little bag and your packed lunch. And I feel so helpless. I just want to grab you up and give you a hug before you go in there but we can't.'

I shrugged. 'That's how it is.' When I walked in, I thought, I can't believe this is happening again.

I had to ask a porter where the oncology day unit was and after all the initial temperature checks and what have you for Covid was done, I went, here we go again, let's get this thing done and over with.

The ward was bigger than I'd expected and contained these captain's chairs that recline. There were tables and non-reclining armchairs too.

There was a haematology ward next door, which had beds that you could book to lie on and sleep while you had your treatment.

It was done out all very nicely and they had a lovely guy who came around with tea and biscuits, and at lunchtime we were offered a sandwich.

Of course, with Covid-19 it was difficult to do things, in that you couldn't be close to anybody and the nurses were all covered in PPE and masks, which they needed to protect themselves from us, but also to protect patients' immune systems as they were so low.

Anne went in earlier than me because she was having anti-sickness drugs first, and when I walked into the chemo ward, she was all wired up with a cannula in each arm.

'What's that about then?' I asked her.

'That one in my left arm is for emergencies if I have a reaction or something happens or they need another line, then they've got that one in.'

'Oh, you will be fine, Anne; don't panic,' I told her. 'I'm actually so glad we're doing this together.'

The nurses put us in chairs side by side and we chatted away about this and that but after a few minutes Anne started to turn purple. I mean, it happened so quickly, and she looked like her head was going to burst open.

'I don't feel right, can you call the nurse?'

I turned to shout help! But the medics had spotted her. One of the nurses shouted, 'Reaction!', and about six of them rushed over and in her spare arm where she had the other cannula, they pumped through a jug load of steroids and other stuff in it to flush it all out.

They were brilliant and work so fast in these situations.

They literally look around, shout reaction and everybody just drops what they're doing. It was like a disaster movie.

Of course, I'm sitting there thinking, I'm next, you know? Geez, I could die here.

Anne's face and head had returned to normal colour, but she looked terrified by the whole experience and I don't blame her. She offered to wait with me, while I finished mine, but I told her to go home with Maureen and rest up.

After her allergic reaction to chemo, Maureen messaged me to tell me that Anne wanted to get in touch with me and to call her back. When I did call up, she was just crying down the phone, saying, 'I wish you were here.'

That meant so much to me and I said, 'You know, Anne, I will sanitise hands, wear a mask and stand at the door, whatever you need.'

She was so scared that she'd had this kind of reaction to chemo and her anxiety was all over the place but just that sentence – I wish you were here with me – was so important to me and I would do anything for her.

My chemo was palliative so a different strength to Anne's. It was called Abraxane – to treat breast cancer that has spread to other parts of the body – which I had every three weeks for six weeks. And Anne ended up being put on it.

This chemo is the one that gives us the pins and needles and horrible side effects. My feet wake me up in the night the pain in them is that bad. It's the worst pain I have endured throughout my cancer – worse than the pain of my mastectomy – and I have to live with it, but it's hard. I am going to try acupuncture to see if that can alleviate any of the discomfit. Another side effect is difficulty speaking and it sounds like I'm drunk, sadly I am not!

The next week I went in again for my chemo session one of the nurses came across to tell me that Anne had had another allergic reaction.

'Oh no!' I panicked and looked over to see Anne in serious conversation with her consultant, Mr Bezecny, tall, thin, wears glasses, who was discussing trying another kind of chemo on her.

I walked over and chuckled to myself when I heard Anne tell him, 'You're killing me.' He replied, 'No, cancer is killing you.'

Mr Bezecny and I first met in 2017 after my fall and the discovery that my cancer had become metastatic. My first impression was that he was not very chatty or good at putting you at ease kind of thing.

But Anne loves him and thinks he's really funny. And that if I'd got to know him, maybe it would be the same.

He gave a stern warning over Covid, saying that because I was in the high-risk group anyway, because of my age and because they were decreasing my immune system through the chemo, if I got Covid I would die.

I mean I understand he has to relay warnings over Covid but I was quite shocked by it and felt he might have said it more sensitively.

Anne was not in the least offended and loves him. But I don't think he would be good for me. I need somebody with a gentler touch.

Mr Danwata has got a lovely smile that brightens up the whole room. And he's really nice and caring; he puts you at ease. I remember him saying to me when he watched a TV show of me receiving my results from when I was under his care in 2017 that I had made him think about how traumatic it was for people hearing their results and having their lives changed forever. He said watching himself on the show reminded him that while it might be his 16th patient of the day he is speaking to, he is about to tell them something that might change their lives forever and that every patient he sees is treated with complete compassion and care.

And he has carried that kindness through all his dealings with me. He makes you think you're the only person he's treating and that you matter to him, which is what I need – to feel taken care of by them.

I had told Anne that when you have chemo, you make friends that you'll never see again, and you get to know people as they come and go, including the nurses. They are literally called chemo mates.

There were all kinds of characters in our ward.

There was this one woman across from us who said, 'Excuse me, are you Linda Nolan?'

I said yes, and she went, 'Oh my God.' And she began to do the hands, like I'm not worthy sign.

It was my turn then to think 'Oh my God.'

Then she recognised Anne and started asking lots of questions.

She told us she and her boyfriend were big fans, which was lovely to hear, and we liked talking to her, but then she got her phone out to take a picture. Fortunately, I didn't have to say anything, because one of the nurses clocked the situation and came to the rescue telling her, 'I don't think you should do that,' and to put her phone away. No harm was done and outside of the hospital I would have happily posed for a photo and nattered away but when you are in that situation you don't want to have to be on guard about what you say and what you do, just because somebody's nice to you. They might hear something and tell somebody else. I'm a chilled person who loves to talk to anybody whether they are or aren't a fan but that was one thing we didn't want to have to deal with, on top of everything else. You just don't act like that around sick people dealing with cancer; when you see them you give them their privacy and space.

Of course, there were lovely people too. People sent cards, addressed to the Nolan sisters, care of Blackpool Victoria Hospital. The nurse joked there was so many they would have to create a bigger pigeonhole for them. Every time we went in, we'd be handed four or five cards from our lovely fans and it was heart-warming reading them. It gave us the motivation to keep going, knowing so many people cared and were behind us willing us to get better.

Fans also told us we were an inspiration, or would write, you are the reason I checked myself and found out I had cancer or, you've inspired me all through your journey.

It was heart-warming to read their many lovely messages and to know our struggles are shared by so many others and that you are helping them by showing them how you're handling it. That helped me to feel strong.

Another girl I follow on Facebook sent me a voucher for a full body massage in Blackpool, because she saw on the show we did how much I enjoyed my massage on the ship – so incredibly thoughtful of her and these kind gestures from strangers meant the world to me and helped me to keep going because I knew it was helping them.

Things didn't get off to an easy start for my first chemo session because they couldn't get the cannula into my arm. And they got me some hot water to put it in to try and flush it through.

I'm sat there going, 'No pressure, but this is the only arm you can use because my left arm is out of use due to lymphoedema!'

Anyway, three of them said they were going to get Tricky Dicky – Richard was a nurse there – because he could, to quote them, 'get them in any vein.'

It had been a long time since I had a needle in my arm and Tricky Dicky struggled too with inserting it. He had red hair and was lovely – very chatty and talked really loudly. The banter was good among all the nurses on the ward.

'What's going to happen now?' I asked.

'We're going to give you a PICC line,' he announced, and he explained it would be an entry point on another place in my body, which would be with me permanently until my chemo was completed, to make things easier for me as I wouldn't have this palaver every time that I came in. All they would need to do is attach the bag to that, and I would carry on my treatment as normal.

They fitted it and did a flush through to check it was working. Bingo! Next was an anti-sickness drug, which takes 20 minutes to kick in, followed by the chemo itself, which takes 40 minutes. Then there was some more waiting, before another lot of chemo is slowly dripped through.

Denise had packed me with enough food for the whole ward. So we had tangerines and chocolate biscuits.

She'd also put a water bottle in and a box specifically filled with gifts for people starting breast cancer treatment, which contained a lovely neck pillow and a beautiful blanket, colouring books, which are great just to take your mind off things when you're unable to switch off, and ginger sweets for the nausea.

In the past, the girls would come in to visit me during a session and bring me in a sandwich, or something like a chicken salad or some hot food, but that was all stopped due to the pandemic. Suddenly you're completely on your own – Anne and I weren't, because we had each other, but for the other poor people it was a tough time.

When my first treatment was done, I felt no allergic reaction like Anne had, much to my relief, and I went out to meet Maureen, who was waiting with the car outside to take me back home to Denise's for my three-week break between sessions. She went back later to collect Anne, and we said, right, we've started the 18-week-long chemo cycle. One session down, five more to go.

That first night I felt okay, but then the dreaded after effects would creep up on me and I used to spend about three days in bed. The first time I spent five days in my bed, and I was that bad

I didn't eat, I just slept all day and night. All my taste buds were gone and even keeping down water was a struggle, and I had to force myself to swallow it.

I hate to use the word journey, but sometimes it's the most accurate way to describe what we were on – a journey dealing with cancer.

Five days after every chemo session, I had to have an injection into my stomach to stop blood clots forming. The district nurse came to do them at about three o'clock on the Saturday – our chemo sessions were always on the Friday.

Well, after my third session, the nurse had been and gone and I was sitting down watching the television. I suddenly said to Denise, 'Oh God.' She asked what was wrong, and I went, 'I have more pains in the bones in my legs.'

The pain was horrendous; I would describe it as really achy like flu. I said I was going up to bed and I tried to get to sleep but I couldn't get comfortable, as the pain was so agonising.

I couldn't remember such a feeling from the first time I had chemotherapy in 2006.

About midnight I said I couldn't take much more of this and I called the 24-hour helpline number we had been given. One of the nurses came on and I told her I was sitting on the edge of my bed, crying from the pain. I'd taken paracetamol but it hadn't touched the sides. They arranged a prescription for co-codamol and Tommy, Denise's husband, drove to the all-night pharmacy to collect it. That didn't touch the pain either and I just cried all night.

The next day the pain was growing worse. I think it was my knee swelling, which was classed as one of the serious side effects. This, combined with bleeding at the PICC line feeding site, a low number of white cells, diarrhoea, constipation, loss of appetite, sore mouth, hair loss, tingling of the hands and feet, tiredness, heart rate changes – the list was endless, and Anne and I had it all. However, the bone pain just exacerbated it all, and I was in constant agony. Eventually they said I could go on morphine and issued Oramorph, which is a liquid form that gets to work fast. Now I'm taking morphine tablets.

I was on 10 milligrams, then 15, 20, and eventually went up to 30 milligrams twice a day, slow release, which gives me constant pain relief for 12 hours a day and makes such a difference.

In September I started to deteriorate and was suffering with breathing troubles. Whenever I breathed in my chest felt like it had been squeezed in half and I couldn't get enough air into the space left in my lungs.

It continued hurting and I felt short of breath even just sitting down doing nothing. I think everybody suspected it was coronavirus because of the nature of the symptoms. I was rushed into hospital where it was discovered I had pneumonia - inflammation of the lungs.

I panicked at hearing the word pneumonia because it brought images of somebody in an oxygen tent and I thought has it been caused by coronavirus because it is a respiratory disease? And will I end up on a ventilator struggling to breathe?

I was tested and thankfully found to not have coronavirus, but I was taken into another ward in isolation for a week to treat the pneumonia and the seriousness of the situation was not lost on me. Pneumonia can be very dangerous, but even more so in immune compromised patients such as myself. Please let me get better I prayed. I haven't gone through all this chemo to throw in the towel at this.

My lungs felt like they were being compressed by an iron band around my chest and all I wanted to do was sleep. As well as dealing with the pain and fear of being so poorly, it was also hard being on my own, away from everybody, while they pumped lots of antibiotics into me. I lay there in tears panicking at the situation and my family cried and worried too.

There were some dark moments lying in the hospital bed where I wondered would I even wake up in the morning, let alone see my family and loved ones again, but with the brilliant medical care I received I began to slowly recover and get a little stronger each day. After a few weeks I was deemed well enough and strong enough to be released from hospital and be allowed to continue my chemo.

Anne had started her chemo before me and so she finished before me last August and marked being discharged from her treatment by ringing the cancer bell at the end of the ward.

Ringing the bell at the end of cancer treatment is a symbolic tradition and it felt incredible and inspiring she had reached the amazing milestone, so I was thrilled when I saw Anne pull the cord. She has come through such a personal battle, not just with her cancer but also with crippling anxiety made worse by the horrible reactions to the first lot of chemo and going through the double nightmare of dealing with it all during a pandemic.

It felt like I was ringing it too watching her take that last walk through the ward to the exit, even though my own journey at that point was still not over.

When I myself got to go and ring it, it was a fantastic feeling, and I was overcome by emotion. In ceremonial tradition the nurses all came out and cheered me and I felt invincible when I walked out the ward and was looking forward to getting my life back.

All felt good initially and I prayed like Anne, who was cancer free, that the chemo had done its work on me. A few weeks later I was sent for an MRI to check the cancer had been blasted. I do hate them as the machine makes me claustrophobic but needs must and as it was my liver they were scanning they said they'd put me in the machine feet first – a much more pleasant way of doing it.

Sadly, I didn't get the news I was looking for from the results of the MRI.

The scan showed it had spread and another tumour had grown in the liver. I burst into tears again at the news, which, when it was delivered this time, was made more difficult by Covid raging again and from being socially distanced from my entire family at a time when all I wanted was a massive hug from them all.

And so my chemotherapy treatment continues to this day. Thankfully, I don't have to keep going into the hospital every three weeks but can take the chemotherapy in tablet form. I have ten tablets a day – five in the morning and five at night and if you were to shake me you would hear me rattle!

I try to find ways to make light of the situation, but it's not pleasant and all the side effects are pretty much still there, but it is a big step from being stuck in a chair wired up to a bag, with cold liquid pumping into your body, burning your veins. But while I do try and downplay it, I have my dark moments where I think about dying and what happens afterwards, and I get scared. I hope there is somewhere we go to where I can see Brian and Bernie once again.

ANNE

It was very different this time round in comparison to the first time I'd had chemotherapy 20 years earlier. We had our temperature taken at the door before we actually went into the unit, then when deemed safe and checked for coughs, the receptionist put a wristband on us and told us we could go through. I had my first chemo session on my own because Linda didn't start until a week after me. I walked in and it wasn't awful. It was quite a nice room actually, pleasant décor and everything was set up to be socially distanced.

In previous times you were allowed to bring somebody with you but that was all hit on the head due to Covid rules.

A nurse asked my name and sat me down and they were so lovely, but this time I couldn't help but notice they all looked really young as well or was it that I am getting old? The first thing they did was start asking me questions and then they asked about using my veins for the cannula.

Fortunately, I have good veins, so they didn't have any problems with that. Needless to say (pardon the pun!), they did end up with them as we went on because my veins started collapsing.

I brought my little radio to listen to music and my Kindle to read, because I knew I'd be in there all day from 9am to six in the evening.

In actual fact I was there till about eight o'clock that night because it was my first time and I was having different lots of treatment.

You're allowed to get up and make yourself a tea, and they come around with a trolley, and you get a sandwich at lunchtime and then a cup of tea and a biscuit.

They've got comfy grandad chairs with bottoms that come out at the flip of a switch, so you put your feet on them, and normal armchairs too.

And they've got all these machines with bags hanging from them, with people sitting around hooked up to them. Most people were sitting there, either reading or having a snooze, or eating or watching other people as well.

The nurses wore visors, which felt surreal; they looked like something out of space with all the PPE and they were always very busy with their hands full rushing back and forth from patient to patient. Despite the pressure they were so lovely and were always asking, 'Is everything okay?'

I was tired by the end of it because I'd been stuck in the chair for the best part of half a day. Maureen came and picked me up and I was relieved that the first session was over, and said to them all, 'see you in three weeks.'

I didn't feel ill the next day either.

The tiredness and sickness hit about three days later. They tell you that the first week you'll be ill and then the second week you should be feeling much better and by the third week you'll be just back to your old self when you come back in for more chemo. But

I was never back to my old self. Even when I went back to the next session of chemo, I didn't feel like my old self or 100 per cent. As the days went on, I started to have quite a bit of nausea. I didn't vomit or anything, but my body felt absolutely wiped out. I also had no energy and I suffered really bad anxiety, so spent most of the time in bed. I also was frightened of going out because of the virus, because I'd been told by the medics in no uncertain terms that if I contracted it, it was curtains for me, so that scared me from going outdoors. I would either sleep or spend the time in bed doing crosswords, watching TV, reading books. I watched all of *Homeland* and *Suits* during my treatment protocol and loved both shows.

But going to the unit itself wasn't horrendous. They were just so nice. You just sit there, and they put a needle in you and you have to be patient as the hours tick by.

It was very clinical there, although at one point it was somebody's birthday. All the nurses had bought a present, and they got together in the middle of the unit and gave it to her, then brought out a cake and we all sang 'Happy Birthday'.

That was lovely to share as it brought a little bit of normality back.

I also found myself chatting to some of the other patients – stuff about what you were having done, what kind of cancer you had, that kind of thing.

I don't really like talking about health normally especially with strangers, but I did. And then you talked about normal things as well. I met some lovely people including two fabulous elderly ladies, one of whom was almost 83 but she looked 63.

She was amazing. I think it was her third cancer and she was driving herself home after her chemo, which I couldn't believe. I found her strength and determination inspiring.

And then there was this other lady who was coming to the end of her treatment. She told me about the symptoms she'd had during her treatment, such as sepsis. She gave me some brilliant advice, which was that there is light the end of the tunnel; that's what you have to keep in your mind all the time. Even in your darkest days, when you think this is never going away, it will end and there will be light.

I held on to that belief and made sure Linda did too.

It was a treat when they came around the ward with ice cream but a lot of people brought their own food in. Although don't get carried away thinking we were being served afternoon tea on fine bone china; this wasn't the Ritz by any means, but rather a hospital with standard hospital grub.

During my second session I was joined by Linda and I was able to come in later at 11am and finish by 5pm so things were looking up.

Linda started at 11am too, and finished about half three, but she would stay with me till five, which was lovely of her. Having her with me helped a lot because she kept my mind on other things and she brought magazines in and we'd look at them together and natter.

She was positioned two metres from me, but we could still hear each other speak, and it was nice having a loved one nearby. She passed me sweets and she'd bring scones from Denise, or

I would bring scones in, and we would swap food with each other like being kids in school, depending on what Denise and Maureen had conjured up for our lunchboxes that day.

Linda was the one who labelled us the Chemo Sisters and I love that moniker.

She's really extrovert and talks to everybody. She chats away and finds out who they are and what they're doing. By the end of it she had all the nurses' phone numbers in her phone and knows all their names, whereas I'd only memorised a few.

She just made life much easier.

The only time I saw my oncologist was when I had that reaction to the chemo, and he had to issue another chemo for me; otherwise the nurses did everything such as administering the drugs, and monitoring the stats. There's a 24-hour helpline so that if you go home and get anxious, or in case you have strange symptoms, you can call and speak to a doctor, even if it's four in the morning. I must have drove them mad because I was always phoning them up.

I got better as I went on, but because of the reaction I had every time I noticed something different, I froze with fear, then my mind would start whirring with all the things it could be, and I would ring up and ask why it was happening. Like when I first developed neuropathy. I got pins and needles in my fingers and my toes, which I knew could be a side effect, but then I started getting what I can only describe as sunburn. It felt like someone had burned the skin on my arms, my face, around the back of my neck and my head, and I thought, what the hell is this? This isn't pins and needles. So, I phoned them up and they told me it sounded also like neuropathy, which was making my nerve endings burn.

They said I needed tests and I spent a whole nine hours being scanned and having ECG tests … everything they could think of. Turns out my anxiety was exacerbating the side effects of the chemo.

Linda had similar side effects to me, and we would talk our symptoms through with each other, as well as our coping mechanisms, and it made me feel better knowing I wasn't the only one going through this and that I wasn't alone.

We chatted about day-to-day things too, be it some celebrity or what we were going to watch on Netflix; because of the pandemic you couldn't do much other than watch TV or read. We'd give each other our TV recommendations, or chat about what the kids were up to, and the decimation of theatres and the arts with the pandemic, how entertainers and performers were getting treated badly, and how it's nearly crippled our industry.

But sometimes she'd be sitting there chatting to me about something and I'd nod off. I'm sure I snored too, because one time I went home to my sister Denise's house, and I fell asleep on the couch. When I woke up, they were all laughing and said 'you've been snoring!'

I said I didn't snore, and they laughed and went, you do!

The second chemo session was when catastrophe struck.

The chemo that was being pumped into me was called Docetaxel. I was just sitting there, only about four or five minutes into the treatment, chatting, laughing on, and joking about things, when I started to get horrendous pain in my lower back and my legs, and my heart was racing. Palpitations and I just thought, my God, something's happening. And I shouted to the nurses, 'HELP!'

My face felt on fire – it turned purple like a blueberry and within seconds a team was around me, taking the intravenous needle out and then pumping other stuff into the cannula to counteract it. And within less than a minute, all the reaction started to go away, and I was back to feeling normal.

Of course, when those scary incidents happen you worry about it happening again, and I nearly said no more treatment, but my oncologist put me on another drug to see how I would fare on something different.

However, I had a reaction again, and this time it was kind of worse because the first thing I noticed was flashing lights in front of my eyes, and I shouted, 'Reaction happening again!'

With this one I also got the pain in my lower back again and in my legs, and my heart rate was racing then started to fall.

This time they brought a specialist team of young doctors down who did an ECG on my heart and made sure that it was all right.

I started to wonder if I was allergic to all chemotherapy, but my oncologist did his work and mixed me up a new prescription, replacing the Docetaxel with a different one called Abraxane, which is the one that Linda was having. I was also taking Carbo-platin and so those combined were what I took for the remaining sessions. I was okay with them although I still had some unpleasant side effects.

I did have days where I felt a little bit better, but never days when I felt back to my old self. The neuropathy and the sunburn feeling didn't grow any worse but it can be very painful and even now I suffer with tingles in my feet and sometimes my hands and I feel I'm walking on eggshells and my fingers tingle and pulsate.

It's a horrible sensation but I have learned to live with it and can deal with it as it's not pain as such, whereas Linda has to really mentally push herself through the pain it causes her.

Mr Bezecny prescribed an anxiety tablet to help overcome my fear of the chemo and relax me while I was having it. He's an amazing doctor and I liked his straight way of giving you an answer. He's very laid-back and dry, and you can have a laugh and a joke with him. I liked his attitude towards things and he never got cross at all my questions. You knew he was giving you an honest answer.

One of the nurses I remembered was called Vicky and she was lovely. She came and sat with me and chatted to me about alternative stuff that was safe to try and could be used alongside the NHS protocol.

She left to go to another unit, but we keep in touch and she texts from time to time to see how I am, and we've been for a socially distanced coffee.

There was also a lovely Chinese nurse who was fascinating to talk to when she would hook me up. I used to ask her endless questions about China and she would talk away. It was like a free history lesson and I learned a lot from listening to her – all the different foods and about the language. I would like to visit China when all this virus has gone.

All the nurses were fabulous and lovely. Kate, who administers the Herceptin that I have to continue to take every three weeks, needs a mention as she is so patient and respectful of my anxiety and needs.

There was a really young junior nurse too on the ward called Abby, who made you feel like a friend, remembering your name and putting you at ease. She was so gentle and never made you feel like you were being a pain. And I know sometimes I maybe was a pain because of my anxiety, asking them all kinds of questions and just worrying unnecessarily when they were trying to give me my treatment.

When it came time to ring the bell, I was thrilled. The bell is at the end of the ward and you ring it to demonstrate you've made it through your treatment.

I didn't feel I had come through unscathed, because while I had finished my chemo in August, I hadn't finished with cancer yet – you still have five years before you are discharged from cancer.

But I did feel very proud that I'd pushed past the side effects to get to the end as chemo is the biggest thing to deal with while you are going through cancer stopping you from living life the way you want to live it and making you feel sick. It was fantastic feeling that I had finished with chemo but I really rang the bell hard for Linda and was doing it for her rather than for me.

My latest scan has shown the cancer has been annihilated, which was the best news possible for 2021, and now my treatment protocol is a preventative one.

I'm currently taking Herceptin every three weeks for the next year. I do think it causes a lot of my side effects but it's helping to keep the cancer at bay. I'm also taking a treatment to prevent the cancer coming back in the bones, called zoledronic acid. I have to take that every six months for the next three years.

The problem with these tablets is that they've all got bloody side effects, but I suppose every drug you take has got a side effect.

It doesn't necessarily say I'm going to get the side effects, but knowing my bloody body, I probably will.

Some of the side effects of zoledronic acid are particularly nasty and can affect your bone marrow and be very painful. I had to make an appointment with my dentist before I took it to make sure that my jaw is in good nick and my teeth are healthy.

My doctor said I didn't have to take zoledronic acid, such are its powerful side effects, but 'I would recommend that you do.'

Maureen was with me when I went to see him and she said, 'You've got to have it; the pros outweigh the cons,' so I am taking it.

My job now is to be there for Linda as she goes through this next chapter of treatment, as she was for me.

CHAPTER 11

FAMILY TIES

ANNE

In Ireland, every name has a meaning, and every family has a motto. Nolan means noble and famous, and our family motto is 'one heart, one way', which to me is gorgeous and perfect for our family because for all of us in the family it really is one heart, one way.

I have a plaque made from Connemara marble, which has our motto and our family crest carved into it. It hangs in my hallway and every day when I went out the door to go to the hospital it gave me the strength to keep going during the dark days of chemotherapy.

Our diagnoses not only changed our individual worlds, but they also changed the worlds of our family. Denise cared for Linda at her home, so her life changed. She had somebody else in the house 24/7 that she wasn't used to. And Maureen actually moved out of her house and into my home to help me out, which was life-changing for her as well. She had times she couldn't see her grandchildren even when lockdown had been lifted because I was shielding and there couldn't be any risk of contact with people because of the fear of contracting Covid-19.

Not only were we battling cancer but Covid also affected the rest of our families and impacted all of us in various ways. They couldn't come to see me or Linda because we were vulnerable, they weren't allowed into hospital with us, and we had to stay in our bubble.

We just got on with it as best we could because what choice did we have? However, dealing with a life-threatening illness during a worldwide pandemic is a lot worse than it could be. As well as our family having to deal with Covid, they were having to do so while two of their family had a life-threatening disease. Despite it also being very difficult for them to go through, everybody's been positive and just getting on with it as best they can.

There have been times I've been feeling up to going out and so has Linda, and when we have been able to get out, we've done things that we're allowed to do with regards to Covid as well as our illness, and our family has been amazing helping us do that.

They have done this by making sacrifices so we can be somewhere that maybe they don't even want to be. They have just been amazing, and if I didn't have my family, I don't know what would have happened.

This book for me has been a chance to say thank you to my amazing family. We have had lots of ups and downs over the years and it's easy to take your family for granted until something like this happens, and then you realise how important they are to you.

I mean, how would I have coped without Maureen who ran me to hospital and has cooked my meals, washed and ironed my clothes and cared for me? I know my daughters would have been there for me, and they have both been fantastic – the most loving and caring daughters a mother could wish for – but they've got their own children to look after and jobs to hold down too.

My family have been such a comfort and joy to me. My girls have been so supportive – I can phone them up crying and they calm me down, telling me: 'You know, Mum, it's your chemo making you feel like this' or 'You're going to be fine'.

'You're being brave', they keep saying, when I don't believe I'm brave at all because I'm just doing something we have to do. A brave person is a person doing something that they don't have to do, such as a fireman rescuing others from a burning building putting his own life at risk or somebody jumping in a fast-flowing river to pull out a drowning person. I have an illness with two choices – I can get better if I take all the medicine with its horrible side effects, or I can decide not to do anything and let nature take its course. But making that choice doesn't make me a brave person.

I'm so proud of my daughters and the grandchildren they have given me. They don't pull any punches and they keep me in the present moment. My granddaughter told me: 'I don't like you without any hair, Gran, but I still love you because you're my gran'.

My eldest grandson is just divine. He just turned 11 last year and is the most gorgeous, beautiful child; he's like a tonic.

My special mention goes to Linda, with whom I have this special unique bond now for the rest of my life. When you go through something like this with somebody else, it cements you together and you become solid as you are going through it. Sometimes we can answer for each other when it comes to talking about the cancer because we've been side by side all the way and know almost what the other is thinking and feeling. Being able to talk about it to her and just knowing that she's there makes all the difference. I can call her and ask questions and she's not going to be put off; she will know the answers to those questions or know how I am really feeling because she is going through the same thing. I can't imagine going through this process on my own and don't know how I did so the first time.

I remember we had gone out together to lunch with the rest of the family when we were chatting and we both started stuttering at the same time due to the chemo side effects. We both looked at each other and knew nobody else probably even really noticed our broken speech, but we knew what that was about. And now I'll see her sometimes rubbing her fingers and I know it is because they're tingling, and I understand the frustrating painful sensation she is feeling because I have suffered with it too. The others are amazing but, because they're not going through that process, there are some things that only Linda will get and understand when I talk about them.

Likewise, if she is struggling to say something because of the stuttering, I know what she means and can step in and say it for her. The stuttering is horrendous, and it can be embarrassing when you're out in company. I tell her the best thing to do is to say to people: I'm so sorry I'm stuttering; it's part of the chemo.

It's interesting how family dynamics change and evolve over the years; growing up with our age gap I didn't see as much of Linda then.

Linda is very chatty, she always has been, just as Bernie was, and is very extrovert. We are complete opposites. She will talk for Britain, and sometimes I think I can't be bothered trying to get a word in, which I don't mind because I like to listen to other people and enjoy Linda's chatter. I'm not an introvert by any means, but I'm quiet; I listen rather than talk. Even when all my sisters are together, the five of us would be all talking at the same time, but at some point in our conversation, I will just sit back to listen and let them get on with doing all the talking.

I'm like that with my groups of friends too. I've had a best friend for almost 60 years – Jackie. We went to school together, and she is a talker and I'm a listener, which is great as that dynamic works brilliantly for us. It's as intense as my relationship with my sisters.

When I was a teenager, she gave me my first bra because my parents were very strict, and I was very shy, and I would never go to my mum and tell her that I needed to wear a bra. Jackie stepped into that role and was the person to give me my first bra and my first pair of tights, bringing them into school for me. I'm just so close to her, as I am to my sisters but it's a different kind of relationship, because with my sisters we've been together since we were born, we share blood. Jackie wasn't with me when Denise and Maureen were born, but she was with me when Linda, Bernie and Coleen were born – an extension of my sisters in a way.

My two brothers Brian and Tommy and their families have also been great. My sisters are more hands-on than the men, but my brothers are in contact and will regularly text me asking me if I want any shopping done, and they'll do it if I ask them.

We have two family WhatsApp chats – one for the sisters only and another for our brothers and extended family. We're practically on those chats all day, every day, sending each other funny pictures, and there's no room for feeling down when you look at all the endless messages of support and memes to make you laugh back and forth.

LINDA

The Cavalry as Brian nicknamed us has always been close but after what Anne and I have been through as a family we are united.

I would never be scared to ask for help these days the way I was after Brian died.

Denise and Tom have been utterly amazing. They opened their doors to me while I was embarking on a new chemotherapy treatment and have gone above and beyond.

It was great for me to get back to my home in time for Christmas and be with my little dog baby Betsy, and, although they never said it, I'm sure they like having their space back as well.

Maureen, Coleen and my brothers have also been lifesavers, and no task has been too much trouble for them, like driving me to appointments, picking things up and just listening when I have wanted to have a cry.

Lockdown has given us all an opportunity to slow down and spend real quality time with each other without all the various distractions.

But my partner on this strange journey in 2020 has been Anne. I was feeling so much closer to her already before this, during our cruise, but sharing our battle to beat cancer together has bonded us in an unbreakable way.

We have been swapping tips all throughout the year. I also recommended a therapist to her to help her combat her anxiety, which has been really good for her, and sent her some self-help books, and she has been a source of strength to me, particularly when the dreaded hair loss kicked off...

CHAPTER 12

HAIR TODAY, GONE TOMORROW

ANNE

With cancer, one of the first things many people ask when they're diagnosed is whether they'll lose their hair.

I understand people asking about that because it's a big thing to lose your hair. It's especially traumatic for women as it's not expected; between the sexes it's seen as an affliction that happens to men as they age.

Not me. Being bald was the least of my problems or concerns when they said I would have chemotherapy.

It's not the worst thing that can happen to you. The cancer is the worst thing. All I cared about was making it through the treatment to the other side.

My attitude was that there are so many other things I'm going to be traumatised about rather than losing my hair, and my hair's going to grow back.

And even if it didn't grow back, I really didn't care. I just thought, it's the least of my problems. I was lucky, you know; I wasn't traumatised by rocking a bald head.

Mine started to fall out between my second and third chemotherapy sessions. I would wake up in the morning and there would be hair covering my pillow and for some reason it was at the end of the bed. I don't know how it got there but when I'd make my bed there would be a nest of hair at the end of the bed to greet me like some weird hair fairy had run her fingers through it while I was sleeping and left it under the sheets and blankets as some sort of hairy gift.

It was getting me down having to clean all this hair up, and when I took a shower more would wash away when I shampooed my head, sliding down my face and clogging the plughole.

Even when I was eating it would fall into my food. Sod this, I thought; I can't be doing this any longer. So, I took matters into my own hands and shaved it all off like Britney Spears the pop star did.

I found it liberating and so much more comfortable without strings of hair making my scalp itch.

Of course, I understand not everybody is like me. You don't have to be bald and show your scalp off if you're not comfortable as there are so many options for women today and men such as wigs, hair replacement services, caps and hats, hats with hair hanging from them, and lovely turbans, which add a glamorous twist to an outfit.

All those choices allow you to pick and choose depending on your mood. For me I was happy to go out bald and couldn't have cared less what strangers thought when I was in the supermarket or on a walk. Let them stare if they want, I thought.

It also saves a fortune in hairdressing bills and you are much quicker in and out the shower in the morning!

The best people to be around when you are bald are children because children don't care. They have the ability to look and say, 'Oh, why don't you have hair?' They don't need to say anything. They just glance at you, clock it, then carry on with what they're doing.

I remember when my grandson played football and I was wearing one of my hats. When I took it off, he went: 'You've actually got no hair.' And I explained that the medicine to make me better makes me lose my hair and he just acknowledged it then went back to playing football. I absolutely adore kids for that.

Linda had a much bigger problem with it than I did. As for millions of others, it was a massive trial for Linda.

When she had it shaved off, she said, 'I won't be going out and I'm staying indoors. I wouldn't going out in public with the bald head, and I'm not wearing those silly scarfs and things.'

Thankfully she has changed her mind. She kind of embraces it now. I mean, I think she still hates it, but now she will go out with or without her cap.

I'm proud of her.

LINDA

Singers in bands get labels, and mine was the blonde with big boobs. I loved my blonde hair; I had nurtured it, held on to most of it the first time around I had cancer, didn't have to worry the second time around, but third time was not so lucky.

The cold cap, which had performed miracles 14 years earlier, sadly was not able to save all my hair from the damage wreaked by chemotherapy due to it not being the right size.

Cancer is a great leveller and it can make people feel lonely. That's why I wanted to go public with my condition to maybe give courage to women out there who are on their own, or who are thinking, I don't want to lose my hair but I don't want to tell anybody that because they'll think I'm vain.

Well, I shouted it from the rooftops. It's not being vain, it's part of your identity. And for women, you know, we can't walk around bald the way a man can because it's not the norm. Hair is part of who we are as women and you shouldn't feel you have to expose that side of things to everybody if you don't wish to. It's normal to want your hair back or to want to wear a wig. You must do whatever makes you feel better until it grows back.

Of course, I was worried about keeping my hair and I tried to wear the cold cap again to preserve my hair while having treatment, but it didn't go to plan.

A young nurse tried to put it on my head but we couldn't get it to fit on properly and it was sticking up around the edges.

I started crying as she moved about trying to stick it down, but I don't think she knew what to do and it wasn't working.

She went to the side of the seat, sat down and just put her hand on mine. 'It could grow back,' she said.

'Oh God, that's not what I want to hear,' I cried. I wanted a solution. I wanted her to do her job and make it fit on or to go and find an alternative not an unhelpful response of 'Oh I'm so sorry the cap doesn't fit, your hair will grow back.'

It's like those first times that people see you bald and compliment your head shape or say, 'your eyes look really big now.' I know they mean well and are trying to be nice, but I know my eyes are already big; they haven't changed shape overnight because you're suddenly hairless.

All I wish is that chemo didn't make your hair fall out to start with. Bad enough you have all the other terrible side effects from the disease and the treatment sending you haywire without also suffering from being bald on top!

That felt a lonely day coming to terms with the fact my hair was going to shortly all fall out and as it started I would walk past a mirror and do a double take because I didn't recognise the person standing in it as my hair grew thinner and more lank by the day.

I'd lie in bed and think about how many hairs I had left. One night I went into the bathroom and I moved the hand mirror around to look at the back of my hair and there were two big bald patches. Nausea washed over me as I panicked: 'What am I going to do? I don't know what to do. My hair is falling out. I'm bald. It's happened.'

Looking back now, I brought more trauma on myself in those first three or four weeks by trying to hang on to my hair, which was never going to happen.

After a certain point it was very obvious my hair was nearly gone and I looked like a fluffy chick, but I was so desperate to try. I would say to the girls, 'I just feel better even with some wispy bits.' As a woman, losing my hair made me feel like I'd lost part of myself: a feeling of being feminine; a feeling of youth.

Apparently when men are told they've got cancer, they ask, will I die? Women ask, will I lose my hair?

It's just such a massive thing for a woman and I found it extremely traumatic. My heart goes out to alopecia sufferers who live with the uncertainty of losing more of their hair and it maybe never regrowing and I would keep reminding myself that one day mine would all come back.

My family were brilliantly supportive, especially Anne who just embraced the Kojak Telly Savalas look and was so brave about the whole thing. I couldn't get on board with it because, like Bernie, I don't do looking like a sick person and being bald everybody automatically assumes you must have some terrible disease such as cancer.

All that was left of my once thick golden waves were little wispy tufts. As ridiculous as I looked, it wasn't easy to let go of them and it took me three times to agree to let my head be shaved, it was that traumatic. I felt stupid having it shaved, and when I rubbed my hand over my head, it felt like Play-Doh plasticine and really cold to the touch.

I was staying with Denise and her partner, and after the last bit was run over with the razor, I walked over to the mirror and took a step back because it was as if Bernie was looking back at me; I was the double image of her. Everybody says that when we were kids they would think we were twins and all a sudden she was there looking straight at me, with this bald head and big blue eyes. It felt weird, and I thought, oh God, here we go again.

Denise asked me how I felt, and I said, 'Well, I've just seen Bernie, I think.'

She said it was because that's how I remembered Bernie at the end of her life, with no hair. She went, 'I'm not being funny, but it looks great.'

I just looked at her in disbelief. Then to wind me up, my brothers told me I have a lovely shape head, knowing how I hated that.

But friends would come in and I knew that they wouldn't know what to say about my bald head. They were devastated for me. I'd ask, 'Have you spoken to the girls?' And they'd tell me they were told not to mention it, to which I'd say it was fine, that I was over it.

Anne was amazing and didn't even bother asking for cold caps; she just shaved hers straight off, no questions asked. She was blasé about the whole thing.

Brian would have been proud of me for going out and about bald. When I first had my chemo in 2006, I'd go to the toilet and he'd get the sticky tape out and pick the hair off the chair I was sitting on or the carpet, so I never had to see it.

But while I still hate it, I have not really bothered with wigs. I will put a hat on instead, although I told my great-nieces and -nephews and grandkids that if my hat blows off down the street, 'Don't be running down there, going there's a bald woman here who needs a hat.'

The doctors put me on steroids for a while and I said to the girls, now I've got a big fat steroid face I look like a boiled egg. You have to find some humour in the situation, or you will cry.

When my hair all grows back in properly after my treatment and is feeling thick and healthy, I'm doing what Bernie did and having it coloured a lovely glamorous platinum.

CHAPTER 13

GETTING WIGGY WITH IT

ANNE

When we went public last year with the story of our joint cancer battle, I was happy to be photographed not wearing a wig. To me it felt honest and natural and this is who I am rather than hiding my scalp behind a hair piece.

In September 2020, we were invited by *Hello!* magazine to do a beautiful shoot about how it felt to ring the bell to signal my chemotherapy coming to an end.

Linda had been struggling with coming to terms with her hair loss, and her making it through the shoot with me was a huge step forward for her in accepting her baldness. She had also just been discharged from a pneumonia battle a day earlier but as ever was a trooper and insisted the show must go on.

Although we both did our best not to show it, the thing that we struggled with that day was exhaustion. Since I'd started having my treatment, I don't think there had been one day where I'd felt 100 per cent or well. Even now I've finished my treatment, I still don't feel well, and Linda also has her bad days where she feels tired and under the weather.

I got up to get ready to go to the hotel for the shoot and my first thought was, Oh God, I don't want to do this – a day of make-up, sorting out costumes, clothes to wear and standing for photographs.

But I thought about how Linda needed this and how it may inspire other women cancer sufferers and once we started the photoshoot, I started to really enjoy myself and I didn't even give my hairlessness a thought.

We had our make-up done by a lovely girl, and then this fantastic stylist came in the room with masses and masses of clothes and was very helpful with styling advice. It felt fun dressing up and messing around and really took my mind off all the trauma.

If we didn't like something, she would find something else fast. I could get used to this royal treatment I thought as she fussed around us both.

I hadn't done anything like this for a long time and I enjoyed trying on all the clothes and feeling the fabrics. Fortunately, the clothes were lovely. I don't wish to sound ungrateful but I have done magazine shoots in the past where the clothes were so frumpy and bad that with risk of sounding like a prima donna, I would end up saying, I'm not wearing any of that!

On this shoot we were even allowed to take a couple of pieces home with us, which was a treat, and the photographer and the assistant were both fabulous, making sure we were okay.

There was a funny episode when Linda and I kept knocking heads and got stuck together – literally. The photographer asked us to put our heads really close together because we both had bald heads. But somehow our heads seemed to glue together – maybe static electricity – and we were saying to each other, I can't move, my head is stuck to yours, and Linda said she could feel my ear in her ear.

We could not stop laughing but it all added to the ambience of it. If you'd come into the room, you would never have thought Linda had a problem with her baldness. She just got on with it with no complaints or tears.

There was another laugh out loud moment when the stylist wedged the pair of us into four-inch high heels. I never was one for wearing heels and we were like newborn foals trying to get up and balance on our legs as we tottered about trying to stay upright, because chemo had kicked us both and sadly left our legs weak and feeling fragile. A stranger staring through the window would have thought we were two old soaks who were drunk as lords as we staggered about hanging on to whatever we could hold that was steady.

Trying to concentrate on the photographer's directions, I could feel my legs about to give way.

'I'm hanging on to you,' I told her while skittering back and forth trying to stay upright. Linda was stronger and stared straight ahead, and, through gritted teeth, said, 'I'm not gonna look at you!' because if she had she would have burst out laughing and we would both have been down on the floor like a pair of skittles.

Our lovely agent Dermot McNamara was on hand to keep an eye on things and check we had everything we needed, and he ordered in afternoon tea and a bottle of bubbly for us. It was a glorious day and Linda and I laughed our heads off.

At the end of it, I said to Linda: 'You look fantastic – the make-up makes your eyes look like bright-blue saucers and you have a lovely shaped head with no bumps. You look beautiful without hair.'

Linda let me get away with saying it to her because I said it with no inflection in my voice and I was telling her the actual truth, which is that she does have a good-shaped head.

My own hair is coming in now and growing back quite rapidly. I've actually got hair on my head now, which has come in speckly grey and black – it looks like a man's beard. But my hairdresser advises me to change the colour to platinum. I am definitely keeping it shorter in length – I don't have time to be worrying about styling my hair.

When Linda was told she would have to carry on with another course of chemo – thankfully from home in tablet form – I did feel guilty my hair has come back in when she misses hers so much, even though that's beyond my control. I do feel sorry for her; I sometimes wish I were still bald so I could be there going through it with her again and Linda didn't feel alone in her suffering.

LINDA

We decided to go to the press because a few journalists had already found out about it and had tried to get in contact with a few of our close friends including my dear Elizabeth Emmett, to check if it was true.

Sadly I lost Liz in February which has been a terrible shock. She was steadfastly loyal and let me know immediately at the time that journalists had called her up asking her 'have the Nolan's got cancer again?'.

It appeared word had got out in the town because we had been spotted at the hospital. I decided to take matters into our own hands and called up our brilliant agent Dermot to ask what should we do. He advised that we take control of the narrative ourselves and give an interview in a newspaper and we decided to go with *The Sun*.

I'd shaved my head two days ahead of the shoot and interview, but I was nervous about being photographed bald for the first time. I arrived at the hotel early, wearing a baseball cap to avoid detection.

I headed upstairs to the bedroom to have my make-up done, and, as we were going up in the lift, our agent Dermot said we were going to do the photos in the bar, and that they'd found an area for us to pose in.

I wasn't comfortable at that point walking around with my bald bonce on show if there were to be loads of people there hanging around in the bar and lounge.

The make-up girl did a lovely job and I never thought in my life I would have make-up applied on my bald head – but I did tell her to make sure I didn't look like a Belisha beacon when I left the room!

Make-up finished, I pulled my cap over my eyes and went down to meet the photographer. I said, 'You don't want me wearing the hat, do you?' He shook his head for no and I went, 'I knew you wouldn't.'

I understood what the score was, so taking a deep breath I thought 'oh, f*** it,' and whipped my cap off. There were only two people in the bar by this point, and one male stranger was lovely. He said, 'Oh, you look fabulous with no hair.'

Anne made a joke about her ears being like pixie ears because there is a little curl at the top of them. And then they wanted me to go up and get a different top, which was fine. But when I got to the actual bedroom, I realised that I'd come up without my hat and nobody had batted an eyelid. I thought, 'Oh my God, how am I going to get down? I'll have to get them to bring my hat up.' However, I braved it and just went down and carried on.

When the story broke in the paper the response was enormous. We were inundated with well wishes from the public and requests for interviews including *Good Morning Britain*. Both of us were asked to take part on a live chat but Anne wasn't well enough to do it, so I had to take the plunge and speak solo.

I did feel nervous, but told myself if I had already got through the first photoshoot with no problems, then I can face the cameras again and talk to a TV studio. I headed back to the very hotel where just a few days earlier I removed my cap and told the world I was fighting cancer.

As I was in the lift to go back downstairs, a lady turned to me and went, 'I saw you this morning on *Good Morning Britain*, I think you and your sister are both amazing. And you both look amazing too.'

There was a funny moment when we were both doing a photograph outside. A bald man walked out the hotel, and I said to him, 'Oh, come on, we can be a trio like Right Said Fred!'

And he said, 'I've read about your story – you're fabulous.'

You know, people are just kind and compassionate when you look back. Initially, I did feel embarrassed about my baldness but that's not through vanity. I know the treatment I am taking that causes my hair loss is to prolong my life but I can still feel really crap about it.

If you get upset because you lose your hair, remember you're not being vain. You can be sad – it is a loss. You have lost part of you. Having gone through it, I find talking about it does help and you have to take the rough with the smooth and try and help other people if you can through it by sharing your own struggles with it.

CHAPTER 14

THREE
SCORE
AND TEN

ANNE

When I was a little girl, 70 sounded so old – an ancient age far away into the future where people required grey hair to show they were wise.

At 17 I thought 30 was old, but when I reached 30, I didn't know why I'd even thought that way.

In my head I don't feel any different at all. It has been the same for every milestone birthday, people always say, 'Gosh, we're going to be fifty. You're going to be forty. You're going to be sixty.'

And when it happens, you honestly don't really feel any different. Well, I don't really feel different. I think it's all a state of mind.

I get more excited about Christmas than I do my birthdays because I absolutely adore Christmas and it's a massive time in our family where we're all together.

I don't think on turning 70 I've changed in any major sense. It's more a case that when somebody asks, how old are you, and I go, '70', I suddenly think, '70, oh God, that sounds so awful' and feel really old.

Also, when my cancer came back, I did initially have a wobble of will I see my 70th?

Well, I made it! That is an achievement and something to celebrate.

My best friend, who I have known since school when we met at 12, turned 70 exactly a week after me, and we both said it is great to reach this age.

I've had such an amazing life as well. The lows as well as the highs are what makes your life what it is.

Turning 70 makes you think about what you have and the things you are grateful for.

Having my daughters and my grandkids obviously is my biggest gift and blessing. And having such an amazing family around me as well through the years – even my extended family of cousins and best friends – who have always been there for me.

My career has also given me a great sense of joy and pleasure. If it hadn't been for being in The Nolans, I would never visited the exotic places I've been, or met some of the amazing people I've met. We weren't a wealthy family, so we'd never have gone to a place like America or Japan or Russia.

We wouldn't have been able to afford it, simply put, but we were given a gift of singing and people wanted to see us and hear us, and it opened doors to all these wonderful opportunities that I might not have otherwise experienced.

When I sit here, I look back and I think, God, I've had an amazing life, and I'm so blessed because not a lot of people have a career like that, as well as children and grandchildren.

My advice to everybody is count your blessings because all your experiences are part of growing older, and what makes us who we are. Try to focus on the good things because they are the things that make you happy and make your life good, not make your life as good as it was. Obviously for me my cancer is going to make a difference but rather than thinking about age I'm just glad I'm alive. And I hope I live till I'm 80.

If I make it to 80 then I will consider myself really lucky that the cancer hasn't got me. When you're diagnosed with cancer, I think the first thing you think is, how long have I got?

I can't speak for other people, but I couldn't help feeling like that, and then you start having a treatment, and you think, I'm going to live, and the question to come into your mindset is, how many more years.

I think about my grandkids; in five years' time my little granddaughter will be 10 and my grandson will be 16, and wouldn't it be amazing to see that?

So, it's not about reaching another milestone but it's about celebrating another year I have had on earth with my family.

Being in the media, I think a lot of emphasis is placed on women looking youthful or following a certain trend. I've never been vain or that bothered about my looks. When we were filming for our television show, they'd say, you need to put more blush on, or you need to put a little bit more lipstick on. And I go, 'Oh, I'm don't really; I'm honestly not bothered.'

I'm not fixated on my appearance and will go out to the shops with no make-up on. And I just think that if I'm just popping to the shop, I'm not putting make-up on just to buy a loaf of bread or something, even if that means people look sometimes.

I'm 70; I don't expect to look younger than I am. My face is a reflection of my life and all I have been through with cancer and surviving it, and if some horrible person was to make a comment about my appearance then it wouldn't bother me if I did hear it. I'd probably think, Oh, that's your problem. Not mine.

The idea of a face lift is not something I would do personally, but not because I have anything against it, or because I think it's wrong. I have no problems at all with women doing what they want to their own bodies, each to their own I think. But I think the big reason *I* wouldn't have it, is because I don't see the point of going through an awful lot of pain when you don't have to.

If extreme bags under the eyes or a big nose and sticking out ears is really spoiling your life and having a detrimental impact on your happiness and wellbeing, absolutely have it done because that's more about mental and medical reasons, but for cosmetic and vanity reasons, it's just not worth the pain or risk, I feel.

I never really had insecurities when I was in school either.

I've embraced my appearance and who I am as a person, and I think that comes from growing older: you stop caring about what others think. And again, I've kind of been blessed in that I've never had a weight problem. I don't know what that would be like to battle with your weight and be on constant diets.

My body is fine, and it doesn't worry me. It's not as new as it used to be and obviously my boobs are not like they were, and I've got veins in my legs and all that, but I just think, so what, I'm 70, you know, this is the process of life and be glad to be alive;

just deal with it. Nobody really cares what you look like and who cares what strangers think?

Perhaps if it did bother me, I might feel different and would go ahead and get stuff done, but for other people, why bother?

My sisters Linda and Maureen have had face surgery because there were things they didn't like when they looked in the mirror. Denise has the same outlook about it as I do. She said, Well, why would I go through all that pain, just to get rid of a few wrinkles, you know? I'm not sure about Coleen, but she's never had any work done. Knowing Bernie, I think she'd probably be along the same lines as me and Denise, but it's hard to say for certain as we never had that conversation.

Men aren't as bothered about appearance as I think some women think or have as many body hang-ups. It does worry me when I see young girls injecting their lips with God knows what to make these big pouty fake-looking pillow lips, which look completely unnatural and will go out of fashion. And if I had my boobs lifted and somebody said to me, 'Oh my God, you look amazing for your age,' I would think, well, actually that is because of surgery not because I have worked hard and worked out all my life to preserve my youth.

You see these stars who are now in their seventies and eighties and they've had masses of surgical work done and people say, oh, so and so looks amazing for her age. Well, she doesn't because she's had masses of work done and you're not seeing what she really looks like for her age because she's worked on preventing that.

Look at the queen instead who is 94, and to me is beautiful. She is somebody who looks great for her age naturally and has embraced ageing – silver hair and everything.

My actual birthday itself was lovely, considering it was in a pandemic. I got up and had messages from all my nieces and nephews and Erin sent me birthday presents in the post.

My house looked like a florist with ten bouquets! I just expected it to pass by, but Maureen made me a lovely breakfast.

We were filming for our show, and she told me that we were filming at Denise's, and when we got there they told me to count to five and then come in, so I guessed there was a surprise awaiting.

When I went in, all of my sisters were there. There was banners everywhere and balloons with all my pictures and pictures of my grandkids on them, which Denise had made, and the table was covered with presents. We opened a bottle of champagne, though I only had one glass because I didn't want to get drunk on camera and be hungover before nightfall.

I was touched by the thought that had gone into my presents. They really were fantastic, and they'd also had a book made, which had messages from lots of friends and family, including Roy Walker.

I had a video message from my dear friend, the late Bobby Ball, which he had composed before he died. We did summer seasons with Bobby and have been close for many years. I got very emotional on seeing that and started to cry. Every time I look at it, I still can't believe he's gone. His death was really sad and sudden, as I didn't even know that he'd gone into hospital. He went in with a chest infection apparently, and it was a shock when his family told us he had passed away.

Sadly, I didn't get to pay tribute and say goodbye to him when he was driven in the cortège through the town, as I wasn't well, but Maureen, Denise and Linda went to stand with the crowds of mourners outside, and his family saw them all wave and knew we were paying our respects. The pandemic stopped him having a normal funeral and I think about how hard it must be for his family, to not have been able to have all their loved ones there and Bobby's many friends and not be able to hug and comfort one another. He was a very great man and I miss him dearly.

After we watched my special birthday video and I opened all my presents, Maureen took me home to rest for about an hour as my sisters were going up to my daughter's house.

I thought, mmm, there are more surprises in store! And then when I got there, Coleen's son, my nephew Shane Jr, was there, which I was thrilled by. He walked me into my daughter's back garden, where my sisters were all there again with my daughters. Coleen had come up from Cheshire too and the biggest surprise was that I was greeted by an inflatable pub in the garden.

It had a little picket fence and a pub sign hanging up, and then there was drinks lined up on the bar. It felt just like a pub.

My daughters brought out a three-tier birthday cake, which had an Arsenal scarf on it because I'm a massive Arsenal supporter, and I was overwhelmed at the effort and trouble everybody had gone to.

My Aunty Theresa was there too, which was wonderful. With her age and with her not being part of the bubble with the rest of the sisters she sat separately from everybody, but despite that aspect it still didn't feel like I was celebrating in a pandemic and it was nice to switch off from all the constant news about Covid.

It was way better than my original birthday party plan pre-Covid, which was for a dinner dance with the ladies in long dresses and the men in tuxes. I turned to my sisters and said: 'This has been far better than anything I had planned because I'm spending time with my closest, favourite and most special people.'

I loved that I could go around the garden talking to everybody without feeling pressure to get around a room speaking to everybody.

The blow-up pub, which the TV company had installed, was fantastic.

Everything was inflated – even the bar seats were inflatables and I had to ask if you could sit on them without them collapsing! The place was decorated with fairy lights and even came with a heater if it got cold.

Shane Jr went behind the bar and was the pub landlord for the day, which he was very good at with his great personality and bags of natural charm, and the grandkids had to ask permission to come in like it was a proper pub.

My young granddaughter found it fascinating and loved sitting in it, drinking a glass of fizzy pop.

It also felt amazing as a family to be together after months of no contact and be in the company of my beautiful grandchildren.

The party went on all day. My daughter has a fire pit in her garden so when it got dark, we sat around the fire, singing songs, which was fabulous fun. I jumped up and I told them, 'Thank you so much for an amazing birthday – I've had the most fantastic time, if not even better than I could ever dream about, and I'm blessed because of what all of you each have done.'

Linda was on great form and let herself go to have a good time. She had a few drinks and was a little bit merry. She loves parties, and being around people gives her such joy. Maureen also let her hair down and had a couple of glasses of Prosecco. I felt slightly inebriated as well.

To sober everyone up, I ordered about 20 pizzas for everybody, which went down a storm. There was no stopping Linda, who was having such a good time, and seeing the time and how late it was I clinked my glass.

Everybody looked at me, waiting for this profound statement to come forth, so imagine their reaction when I told them my daughter is a teacher and has to get the kids to school so last orders were 9.30pm and the pub would be closing at 10pm!

If I had not done that, Linda would still be there now making merry in the garden. She's just like Bernie was – a party animal to the end and always the last one standing.

LINDA

Covid reared its ugly head again when it grew nearer to Anne's 70th birthday, forcing her to abandon her plans for a lovely dinner dance and orchestra.

She was incredibly understanding about the situation and resigned herself to not celebrating, joking she would stay 69 and do it all next year.

But there was no way we were letting that happen. Just as we had for Bernie's In Memoriam 60th, we got to work arranging something for Anne.

Denise organised the banner/balloons with pictures of grand-children, and we planned to stand across the road from her house to sing 'Happy Birthday'. But our TV company production team stepped in and said they would have a think, and, because we were working, we were allowed to have up to six of us indoors on camera socially distanced, so that's what we did.

Denise made a beautiful book with all our messages to Anne. I did a page of pictures of us over the years with all our different hair styles.

The kids just adored the blow-up pub – they thought it was a bouncy castle – and Shane was in his element behind the bar, serving up drinks.

Anne cried all day, she was that happy, and you just wanted to hug her.

The TV company filmed my nieces and nephews saying what they think of me and one said: 'I love Aunty Linda because she lets us stay up until nine o'clock at night and sometimes have midnight feasts of ice cream in bed!'

Sitting around the fire pit, it felt like we were all on holiday together, and I loved being able to sing songs and reminisce with everyone else there.

Anne was appreciative and said it was gorgeous. It's such an achievement getting to 70 anyway, but, to come through what she has come through with cancer and chemo, it was just great to see her there smiling.

I also thought of Bernie, who would have loved celebrating in the pub and singing away with us all. I think she'd have been proud of us.

When I got home that night, I sat there and thought, who is going to do this for me when I die? I'm going to have to leave something in my will – a fiver each to my friends winding them all up to mark my birthday every year when I am no longer here!

CHAPTER 15

GOING FORWARD

ANNE

My seventh decade has taught me a lot. The biggest lesson I've learned is to think before I speak. I still do it sometimes, but I have learned to try and wait and not be so volatile.

When I was younger, if I didn't like something, or somebody said something I disagreed with, I would jump on it. Now I take a step back and think about why they're saying that. Are they depressed, or is this something they really feel strongly about? Then I try to analyse it before I answer and look at it from their point of view. I think that's something I've learned with age, which is a really good thing for me.

When you get older, you learn to appreciate the good things about life, so instead of wasting valuable time thinking, why did that happen?, I try to think about all the good things that I have in life, such as enjoying a beautiful sky, or sitting on the promenade, watching the tide go in and out – those are things I get so much joy from.

If I find myself in a bad mood, I can turn it around by thinking of something I really love. A lot of it is to do with my faith. I'm religious, and I go to mass every Sunday, which now involves watching it on my iPad. My cousin is a priest, and he does the service.

I believe that there is a God above – even though part of my brain tells me I can't believe in something I can't see or feel or touch. I've prayed all through my cancer; I do believe that there is somebody up there listening to me.

When I was ten, I was sent on a pilgrimage to Lourdes, France, because I was in hospital for two years with suspected rheumatic heart fever, but I was never formally diagnosed.

My legs would be in terrible pain and the doctors now say, it's just something you've got to live with. So away I went to Lourdes on my mother's wishes, and when I came back we went to England to be with our family. Mum took me to the hospital in the UK and they couldn't find anything wrong with me. My mum always used to say I was cured at Lourdes. My mum was very religious, and when I pray now I pray to Our Lady of Lourdes and Saint Bernadette. My daughters also have a strong sense of faith and I think they too will have drawn on it like I have in times of trouble.

However, I have had wobbles over the years and I've had lengthy talks with my cousin, the priest, telling him I've had trouble believing at times.

'Ah, but what do you do when you are feeling like this?' he asked.

'I pray,' I told him.

'So that's your faith. Your faith is telling you that there is something there.'

He explained it in such a good way – a way that made me want to continue praying.

There isn't a lot left that I want now from my life apart from time to see my grandkids growing up – that's going to be a great joy to me – and watching my daughters achieving what they want to achieve in their lives. Hopefully they will achieve their dreams, and their lives will be as full as mine has been. I want them all to enjoy long good health their whole lives.

Being a mother was the thing I yearned for the most, followed by good health and happiness. Sadly, lifelong good health hasn't been something I was blessed with, having gone through so much with cancer, but overcoming those battles has made me appreciate even more feeling better and how your own good health is something you should never take for granted.

I have travelled first class on planes, and it does not interest me, nor do designer handbags or being seen at fancy parties or any of the normal trappings of fame, but I would like my own garden and house – my own sanctuary.

Since losing my house in the divorce I have yearned for a beautiful, detached house with a manageable garden to call my own – like the one we used to live in years ago. Even a small bungalow would be wonderful.

These are not lifelong regrets but just a wish, as I have a roof over my head and my grandchildren are everything I could ever have wanted.

I'm not totally without ambition even though I am 70, and I think it's important not to give up on the things you really like and to reach for the stars and follow your dreams and heart.

I got my dream of children and grandchildren, and that's what I'm going to look towards: the things I have in my life and not the things that I haven't had or may never have. Your dreams should never stress you out, but it's good to have them and think, maybe one day... like when people talk about winning the lottery.

Pre-pandemic we would go as a family to the Bingo every week. We didn't always win, but we would go for the camaraderie of a nice night out and have a meal and a drink there.

Through lockdown I think we have all come to realise our time with loved ones is precious and those times as a family at the Bingo are something I really miss, the camaraderie of being together. Being on your own stuck in a house can send you stir-crazy because you start overthinking everything and magnify things that normally would be meaningless into a big deal. When we are busy and getting out the house – be it for exercise or activities, or going to church, or meeting friends and family – you're distracted, and your mind doesn't have time to overthink.

I've actually got a psychologist, recommended by my doctor, to talk to about these things. When she asked me what worries me, I said, 'Well, I'm fighting to stay alive. I don't want to die.'

But I think that's because of the cancer; I've always worried about dying but having cancer makes me think about it and worry about dying much more than I ordinarily would.

My anxiety has improved since seeing the psychologist, and I've stopped taking my anxiety tablets. I'd never before suffered with anxiety despite going through all kinds of things – divorce, nearly dying giving birth to my oldest daughter, fighting cancer in 2000 – but I've never suffered with anxiety, except for this time.

I think what made me so anxious this time is that horrible allergic reaction I suffered to the chemo and then thinking I was going to die from this; it was so fast and all a shock. That coupled with the pandemic being a backdrop – living in fear of catching Covid and dying that that way, fears of Covid taking members of my family or friends, and not being able to hug my family and friends. It's been the most unsettling and upsetting of times but as we ease our way out of a third lockdown and with me now having the vaccine, I think my anxiety is getting better.

My only concern now is getting Linda through this. Her cancer is incurable but it's treatable, and they've told her she could live for another 15 years, so that's what she and all of us are holding on to.

Linda is literally made of Teflon; she has come so far and no matter what she will just keep going. I'm a big believer in the mind as a powerful tool and Linda is the most positive person. Plus, there are new treatments coming out on the market the whole time. She must get through this next round of chemo, which she is thankfully being allowed to do from home with occasional hospital trips to have her bloods done, but we are all behind her, and will help carry her through it just as she has helped to carry me.

LINDA

I really think the cancer has brought us together. Like Anne said, if she can do it, I can do it, and she will be there for me.

Before my last chemo session, when I was on my own, after Anne had rung the bell, she kindly said, 'I will come in and sit with you if you like through yours.' I told her, 'That's so lovely but because of Covid I don't think they will let you in – they're very strict – and mine only takes ninety minutes so I will be home soon. I appreciate that you've offered, though.'

I would never inflict that tedious ordeal on anybody, least of all my sister who had just got through it herself.

We lost our sister-in-law Lindsay 30 years ago, when she was only 26, and since then we've been people who say I love you when we finish a phone call; I think we've all learned that you could lose somebody in a heartbeat. With Anne and me going through a life-threatening illness it is important to let your loved ones know they're loved and appreciated.

Covid has made it all so much more difficult. Without it, our family would have been able to have spent more time together such as Anne and I going somewhere together after our treatment for a bite to eat, or our sisters and brothers being able to swing by our homes, and greet us indoors with a hug and a kiss.

Looking on the bright side, in other ways, though, I would say that cancer has given me a sense of freedom in a way because it has made me prioritise things in the right way. By this I mean that in the past I would feel pressure to take part in things, even when my heart was saying 'no, don't go, there's a million better things you can be doing with your time' and would have an internal battle with myself.

Maybe I struggled back then with being assertive and would say yes to please others instead of pleasing myself. These days I have no such qualms and will happily turn things down because I would much rather be picking up my great-nieces or -nephews from school.

Cancer speeds up your time and you become very aware of how precious every second is.

Hopefully I'm going to be around for a very long time to come, and I will still be here to pick them up as the years go by; however, in case I'm not, I want to make the most of my life now, and that's where it has given me a sense of freedom.

My attitude to life is do it now. If you can do whatever important thing you need to do now, then go and do it. Don't hang around putting it off because you may never get a second chance. Those are some of the ways having incurable cancer makes you take stock of your life.

I'm also better now at expressing my opinion and sticking to it rather than maybe being swayed by others. It all comes down to a question of priorities and what is important in your life. For me that's my family and spending as much time as I have with them.

I have also got back out and started dating. Coleen and I joined dating apps and we both met new people just before the third lockdown. I have been on one date and Coleen has met somebody and been out with him a couple of times, pre-lockdown of course, and Maureen is now talking to somebody online.

It's hilarious, we are like schoolgirls. I set up a sibling WhatsApp group when I got ill so if I wanted to tell them anything I could do it in one go rather than individually messaging them. Coleen went out when we were still in Tier 2 for something to eat and she sent a message afterwards to the group saying, 'I kissed him!' and we were all typing simultaneously 'I'm phoning you to discuss!'

My date before the lockdown was a walk in the park and I was standing there waiting for him to turn up and I said if you are more than five minutes late, I will be gone as I am not standing around like a lemon.

He promised he would be on time saying, 'even if I had to walk, I would get there on time' and I thought oh God don't be too smooth and I had seen a picture of him and it was lovely. We chatted, he brought a treat for the dog and he brought me a pork pie!

I can honestly say I have never been brought a pork pie before. 'Listen, it's not as romantic as flowers but it's tastier,' he told me while handing it over.

He's funny and he's attractive and he sounds like one of Oasis when he talks. Part of me thinks I can't be bothered, why are you worrying so much about dating again and having cancer makes you realise it's not the be all and end all of life. All the what will I wear, where will I go questions you normally have when dating. I was grateful to Covid for taking a lot of those annoying decisions away and I would have been a mortified 12-year-old at school again if he had tried to have kissed me on the first date so Covid helped there too. But he is lovely, and we are still talking and when things are more relaxed and restrictions are lifted, we will meet up for another walk.

ONWARDS
AND
UPWARDS

We said to the others in the family: if you had told us when we were leaving on the cruise in March 2020 that in the space of a year we would do two television series, both be diagnosed with cancer and make it through our treatments while getting through the Covid pandemic and writing a book, we'd have said you were mad. But here we are.

It just shows there's light at the end of the tunnel and everything comes full circle in the end.

People say to us, do you ask, why you? Well, we don't because it was Bernie who said, why not me? There are lots of people who are going through even worse than we're going through. We've seen those who have lost loved ones to Covid-19, and this pandemic is still wreaking havoc on millions of lives.

Our attitude is, how lucky we are to still be here, to be working, to have homes and families who care for us, when so many others find themselves in worse positions.

Sometimes when people tell us that we are fighters, well I think you are all fighters, everyone who is going through this.

We lost Bernie but we carry on for her, soaking up as much from life as we still can, just like she would want us to do, and we're doing okay; we've got our grandkids and nieces and neph-ews, and in that respect, we have to be grateful and remember there are other people out there who are trying just as hard.

We will keep going as long as we're allowed to, supporting each other, for we are stronger together.

Look after yourselves and don't give up.

Anne & Linda x

LINDA'S ACKNOWLEDGMENTS

When I was asked to do this book I said yes, as long as it's accurate and not all doom and gloom. Well, because of you Sarah Robertson I think we have achieved it. Thank you Sarah for making it all so easy, even when it was difficult!

To my amazing agent and manager, Dermot McNamara. Only two (and a bit) years working together and look what you have achieved for me. I could never thank you enough. Your belief in me has turned my life around, the future looks so bright and I'm looking forward to many more adventures with you at the helm!

Anne, what a journey (sorry to use the J word!) we have been on together. You are amazing, and your love and support through all of this have been invaluable. We did it together, I love you X

To all the people out there who have supported me through the years...

Thank you from the bottom of my heart.

A big thank you to all the people below who made it possible for me to tell my story, my way:

Our Publishers Ebury, especially Sara Cywinski, Lydia Ramah and Katherine Josselyn.

Dan Wootton and Victoria Newton. Karen Cross. Siobhan Wykes and Shelley Spadoni. Claire Fitzsimons and Alison Phillips. Neil Thompson. Richard 'Fredi' Frediani.

The wonderful NHS for continuing to look after me, especially my consultant Dr Danwata, breast care nurse specialist Sarah Middleton and consultant clinical psychologist Dr Jean Brigg. I really wouldn't be here without you!

Finally and most importantly my amazing family: Lloyd, Kam and Mia & Gary, Sarah and Lucy. I love you.

My nieces, nephews, great-nieces and great-nephews,

You Are My World.

Tommy & Jackie, Anne, Denise & Tom, Maureen, Brian & Annie, Coleen and Auntie Teresa ... your unconditional love and support is what keeps me going. I love you all so much.

ANNE'S ACKNOWLEDGMENTS

Thanks to the Oncology Unit and the Breast Care Unit at Blackpool Victoria Hospital for the professionalism, kindness, understanding and support. Dr Bezecny my oncologist for being the best there is. Lynnette Bracegirdle my breast care nurse for her kindness and support. Dr Karen Green my psychologist who helped get me through a really bad time during my treatment.

My sister Maureen for giving up living her own life to look after me with love and patience and understanding. My sister Denise for all the thoughtful well needed gifts she gave me and her love and support. Dermot McNamara for providing wonderful opportunities and believing in me. My sister Linda for going through my illness with me and being so supportive and kind. To my sister Coleen and my brothers Brian and Tommy and all my extended family for being there whenever I needed them.

My best friends Jacqui, Joan and Patsy, Adam, Carl and Lee for their caring and support.

To anyone who wrote or texted or emailed with good wishes and prayers.

To Sarah who wrote our story with great empathy and understanding.

And last but most importantly to my daughters Amy and Alex and my grandchildren Vinny, Ryder and Nevaeh, without whose love and support I would never have made it.